Learn About Your Arthritis!

Patients' Guide to Managing the Most Common Rheumatic Illnesses

Written by

Malin Prupas, M.D., F.A.C.P.

HATS
OFF™

International Standard Book Number: 1-58736-028-4
Library of Congress Card Number: 2001116967

Published by Hats Off Books™
610 East Delano Street, Suite 104, Tucson, Arizona 85705, U.S.A.
www.hatsoffbooks.com

Cover and book design by Atilla L. Vékony
Illustrations by Christie Howard

Printed in the United States of America

Acknowledgements I am indebted to several people and groups for the opportunity to write a book about arthritis. The people that have influenced me the most are my patients. Patients taught me many things and never stopped amazing me with their questions, but also their courage and stamina to put up with a problem that rarely went away and was there twenty-four/seven. I am also indebted to my family for all the hours they shared the computer, so I could write down my ideas. They encouraged me often. My office staff helped, including both Deborah Hayhoe and Marsha Feliz proofreading my chapters and making suggestions. They were exceptionally helpful. Physicians and patients made important comments at the beginning of several chapters. Finally, I have been fortunate to have received a great education and opportunities exposing me to many facets of medicine. Books taught me the facts and my professors taught me the skills. It was my parents that stressed the importance of an education, my brother and sister-in-law who helped with the financial burden, and finally personal illnesses with myself and my sister that have helped me realize the importance of it all.

This book is dedicated to the memories of my parents. Both my father and mother always insisted that I be a physician. Although their directions and guidance were crucial to my success, they allowed me to seek out a specialty of medicine that I could master and feel rewarded with. They encouraged me to measure success in inches, rather than miles.

Table of Contents

Introduction

Arthritis is not a silent disease. It growls and roars at its victims. It is easy to understand why victims seek out any help or relief they can find. Because it is so common there is plenty to read about arthritis at the bookstore or even the checkout line of the grocery store. The public is always eager to hear more. At the bookstore you will not only find books about arthritis, but also every treatment imaginable. The tabloids at the grocery store describe the latest diet, exercise, or the newest treatment regime for arthritis. Unfortunately, a number of unproven remedies receive more attention than better-recognized treatments that have either stood the test of time, or have been proven by good clinical studies accepted by scientists and doctors specializing in the care and treatment of arthritis. For the thousands of people each year that develop the first signs and symptoms of arthritis, there are few good sources of information. The lack of concrete and acceptable information about arthritis and its treatment for patients with arthritis has prompted me to write about my twenty years of experience caring for patients with arthritis, and my efforts to make them better informed. This book is intended to fill a void for those who are new to the aches and pains of arthritis and related conditions. Arthritis is a chronic disease that you will have your entire life. Arthritis will affect everyone in the family as a result of the relentless effects of old "Arthur," as it is so commonly called.

Over forty million Americans have some form of arthritis, and one in three families is touched by it.

This text is not intended to replace the guidance and advice of your doctor, but rather to be a supplement and resource for referral. If you happen to read this book first, before consulting with a physician, it is recommended that you do visit your doctor to talk about your further concerns.

The first portion of this book defines the basics of arthritis and rheumatology. Autoimmunity is defined because of its importance in the mechanism of the disease. The major categories of illness are reviewed. There are over 100 types of arthritis now well described. It is neither necessary, nor important to cover all types of arthritis. Many have a common final pathway, the destruction of joints, which interferes with lifestyle and the daily activities of living that so many of us take for granted. For the man or woman whose hands are deformed because of rheumatoid arthritis, holding a coffee cup in the morning is a major ordeal. The second portion of this book is divided by the location of arthritis by body area. The final portions of the book include the answers or responses to frequently asked questions. There is not always a correct answer, nor a best answer, and some will find an answer from their own experiences. Finally, a number of unique situations are clarified, including pregnancy, survival, and disability.

The treatment of arthritis is divided into three categories, including medicine, surgery, and physical and occupational therapies. Alternative treatments are briefly mentioned. One cannot discount the importance of learning as much as possible about all three aspects of treatment. It is crucial that you be an active participant and understand the importance of taking medicine, the natural history of the disease, and disease progression. This understanding will help improve the quality of your life.

Learning new vocabulary words describing arthritis is a useful tool and can provide better communication with you and your doctor or other caregivers. Throughout this book are words that are new and difficult. Medical names, terms, and definitions are not included to be intimidating or impressive, but rather to help give the reader the means to deal with a difficult subject. The subject of arthritis deserves more attention than it has received in the grocery store tabloids.

It is hoped that this book, in some small way will help improve the quality of life for those individuals stricken with arthritis.

Further recommendations and ideas for new chapters, or additions to the vocabulary are always welcome and should be sent to the author.

About the Author The author is a board-certified rheumatologist with over twenty years of experience caring for patients with many forms of arthritis or related conditions. His current responsibilities include acting as the senior rheumatologist with Arthritis Consultants, a group of three rheumatologists in Reno, Nevada, and the medical director of the Osteoporosis Imaging Center of Reno. In addition, Dr. Prupas is an associate clinical professor of medicine at the University of Nevada School of Medicine, and is also board-certified in internal medicine. He is currently a consultant for several major pharmaceutical companies and at this time is conducting multiple clinical drug trials. Over the past 12 years, Dr. Prupas has been the principal investigator for over 50 clinical drug trials of new medicines for the treatment of arthritis. Several of these drugs are currently available and have been approved by the Food and Drug Administration.

The author is an excellent clinician, and has learned to talk to patients and families in a way that instills trust, belief, and hope about an illness that will change the patient's quality of life significantly. Experience has enabled the author to develop thorough, but understandable discussions of most forms of arthritis for patients. In Dr. Prupas's clinic, whether the patient is formally educated or not, each individual patient is allowed to ask questions and leave with a clear understanding of their condition and prognosis along with written handouts about their illness.

This text has been written over the span of several years and is published so that these ideas, concepts, and information learned from previous experiences can be shared with others. Although he has never written a textbook, Dr. Prupas has been published several times by peer review medical journals. Dr. Prupas lectures often to different groups and is always well received.

Dr. Prupas was a member of the charter class of the School of Medicine, University of Nevada, Reno. He transferred to Tufts University School of Medicine, Boston and received his M.D. degree in 1975. The completion of his internal medicine training followed in Southern California. Finally, he completed a fellowship in rheumatology and immunology at USC-LA County Medical Center in 1980, before he relocated with his family to Reno. Dr. Prupas is a Fellow in the American College of Physicians and also a Fellow in the American College of Rheumatology. These organizations are prestigious groups recognizing internal medicine and rheumatology.

Autoimmunity is the basis for many forms of arthritis. The body's immune system normally makes proteins called antibodies that protect the body against viruses, bacteria, and other foreign materials called antigens. In an autoimmune disorder such as lupus, the immune system loses it ability to tell the difference between foreign and its own cells and tissues called "auto" or "self." The immune system incorrectly makes antibodies directed against self. These antibodies, called autoantibodies, react with the self antigens to form immune complexes. The immune complexes deposit in various tissues and create inflammation, injury to tissues, and pain. Over seventy percent of people with systemic lupus have these antibodies deposited in different parts of the body. Several types of arthritis are characterized by autoantibodies in the blood and the immune complexes they form. These blood markers are not foolproof, nor perfect, but serve as helpers in distinguishing disease and activity of disease.

Rheumatology is the medical specialty providing care to people with arthritis and related conditions, primarily disease of the immune system and other disorders that cause pain and inflammation of the joints, muscles, and bones. Osteoarthritis, rheumatoid arthritis, gout, systemic lupus erythematosus, bursitis, back pain, and osteoporosis represent some of the many forms of arthritis or rheumatic illness. Arthritis involves much more than just the joints and can affect multiple other organ systems of the body. People with arthritis frequently receive care not only from rheumatologists who have special training and experience, but also other physicians. People with arthritis are often cared for both by their primary physician and specialists.

Timely consultation with a rheumatologist can help ensure a positive outcome after a prompt and accurate diagnosis and appropriate therapy. Coordinated management by both the primary care physician and specialist is often desirable. A specialist can often diagnose and treat arthritis less expensively than doctors not specifically trained in arthritis management.

Identifying Arthritis

Identifying arthritis can be difficult. Have you ever had an ache or pain and wondered if it could be arthritis or something more serious? Most of the time it isn't arthritis and the ache or pain goes away in a short while. Working in the garden, building the new doghouse, or sometimes just sweeping the driveway can result in a number of aches and pains the following day. The important thing is that these feelings will go away quickly and leave no ill effect. They are a signal of overdoing or straining muscles you haven't used recently. Arthritis is a more serious painful disorder. The pain of arthritis usually lasts longer or returns; it may be one symptom of a more serious disease, and finally there may be evidence of inflammation. If an area is swollen, red, painful, and hot, it is inflamed. This means get help and get relief. Nearly forty million Americans have some form of arthritis. There are more than one hundred different forms of the disease. Arthritis literally means joint inflammation. Unfortunately, most types of arthritis are chronic and last a lifetime. The diagnosis and early management of arthritis is imperative. Early treatment can make a difference! So how do you tell the difference from the aches of pains of overdoing and more serious forms of arthritis? It is crucial that patients with arthritis become educated and get involved in their care. If symptoms last for more than a few days, seem serious, are very painful, associated with inflammation, or recur more than once, see your doctor!

THE MAJOR WARNING SIGNS OF ARTHRITIS

- Swelling in one or several joints
- Early morning stiffness for one hour
- Continual or recurring pain in a joint
- Difficulty moving a joint normally
- Warmth and obvious redness in a joint
- Nodules under the skin
- Joint pain combined with unexplained fever, weakness, weight loss, or rash

---

The following paragraphs describe the most common types of arthritis or rheumatic diseases.

Rheumatoid Arthritis (RA)

RA is symmetrical and occurs on both sides of the body. For example, if one knee is swollen, the other knee may be swollen, per-

haps not at the same time. RA involves many joints and is called a polyarthritis (more than five joints). This form of arthritis primarily affects young and middle-aged women between twenty and forty-five years of age. Men and children are also susceptible to this form of arthritis. The hands are especially involved, but also some of the larger joints like the hips, knees, ankles, shoulders, and elbows. Already, this sounds much more serious than the aches and pains of the weekend gardener. The term "rheumatoid disease" is often used because much more than the joints are affected, including the skin, eyes, heart, muscles, lungs, bones, and nerves. There is a genetic predisposition to this disease, although the details remain to be worked out. The cause is actually unknown. More than one family member may be affected. The joint inflammation tends to be characterized by exacerbations (flares) or periods of inactivity (remissions). The course of the arthritis may appear to be periods of peaks and valleys, that last days, weeks, or months. No one knows what triggers these cycles, but medicine can be effective and provide immediate relief. Rarely, but fortunately, spontaneous remissions occur in some people and the arthritis resolves by itself. If you were to put 100 consecutive individuals at the onset of rheumatoid arthritis in the hospital and follow them closely for an extended time period, a small number would have a short-lived illness that would go away without doing anything, another small number would have a terribly active form of the disease, while those individuals in the middle would have a persistent ongoing illness characterized by continued hot, tender, swollen, and warm joints that develop increasing complications of RA.

Osteoporosis

Osteoporosis is a condition in which bone mass, bone density, and thus bone strength decrease. This results in an increased susceptibility to bone fracture. After menopause the levels of female hormone (estrogen) decrease. The loss of estrogen diminishes the beneficial effects on bone. If estrogen replacement therapy (ERT) is not given during this time, a rapid loss of bone occurs. Bone loss occurs more often in Caucasian and Asian populations. Osteoporosis occurs in association with other diseases and with the use of some medications, especially corticosteroids. Symptoms will not occur until there is an actual fracture, commonly the hip, wrist, or spine (dowager's hump). Bone density measurements done by dual energy x-ray absorptiometry or DEXA are a useful and simple way to look for the risk of fracture and measure treatment effectiveness. Screening DEXA scans are now readily available.

Systemic Lupus Erythematosus (SLE)

Referred to as lupus, this form of arthritis is not uncommon and actually occurs more often than well-publicized illnesses, like multi-

ple sclerosis or leukemia. The disease is characterized by autoimmunity. Antibodies in our body that normally fight infection turn against our "self." This phenomenon can be measured in the blood as the antinuclear antibody (ANA) test. The ANA is found in most individuals with this illness. Usually SLE patients are women of the childbearing ages; however, the very young can be involved, as well as the elderly, or men. About 500,000 Americans between the ages of fifteen and forty have SLE. A small group of people develop this form of arthritis after taking common medications which seem to induce autoimmunity. Think of this illness as a long railroad track. At one end of the track are those individuals who have serious problems, for example involvement of the brain, nerves, or the kidney. At the other end of the track are those people who have less serious or life threatening disease like achy joints or skin rash. Complexes of antibodies can be deposited just about anywhere. The location of the deposited antibodies determines the signs and symptoms of the disease. Symptoms include a photosensitive rash, hair loss, alternating color changes of the fingers, joint pain without swelling, oral ulcers, or a characteristic rash across the bridge of the nose and face.

Fibromyalgia

Fibromyalgia is one of many terms. The illness is also known as fibrositis, myofascial pain syndrome, soft tissue rheumatism, or nonarticular rheumatism. The syndrome includes trigger points that have been well mapped out on the body's surface; poor sleeping habits, and mild depression. There is a vicious cycle of these events associated with marked fatigue. Symptoms can snowball and get much worse. The longer the duration of symptoms the worse the prognosis. People often benefit from antidepressant medication at bedtime to help sleep, knowing more about their illness, and support groups. Many of these people have seen multiple physicians without an answer for their symptoms or have had surgery trying to achieve relief. Alternative health care is actively sought out.

Gout

Many people are not aware that gout is one of the oldest forms of arthritis. Inflammation of the joint is precipitated by a crystal of uric acid. This crystal creates a tremendous response by the body characterized by inflammation and pain. All gout patients have high levels of uric acid in the blood at some time or another, although not necessarily at the time of an acute attack. Therefore, the level of uric acid in the blood should not be used to make the diagnosis. The majority of patients are middle-aged men or postmenopausal women. The first attack usually occurs in the big toe, although this form of arthritis can begin in many joints at once and mimic other forms of arthritis. Attacks begin infrequently, but eventually occur more often and closer together. Treatment includes anti-inflammatory medications during the acute attack. The treatment of the elevated uric acid levels include medications which either help excrete uric acid in the urine or inhibit the formation of uric acid in the blood. The treatment of the uric levels should not be started during an attack, since decreasing the uric level rapidly may precipitate, prolong, or worsen the acute attack. Although there are some important things to avoid while eating, special diets are usually not necessary. Many gout patients are overweight and have high blood pressure or hypertension. Gout patients often come to the doctor's office wearing slippers, cutout shoes or sneakers, or using crutches because they are so uncomfortable. The pain can be excruciating.

Seronegative Spondyloarthropathy

Ankylosing spondylitis (AS) is much more common in men than women and has a special predilection for certain groups. There is a genetic link to the disease greater than any other form of arthritis. Over ninety percent of patients have a genetic marker (HLA-B27) that can be found in a simple blood specimen. This can be confused with about six percent of the normal population who also have the same genetic marker without arthritis. This form of arthritis belongs to a group of illnesses called the seronegative spondyloarthropathies. All of these individuals have a high percentage of positive HLA-B27 genetic markers. Other forms of arthritis in this group include psoriatic arthritis, Reiter's syndrome, and the arthritis associated with inflammatory bowel disease. "Ankylosing" means rigid or stiff, and "spondyl" refers to the spine. "Itis" always means inflammation. The inflammation results in the vertebral bodies of the spine growing together slowly, usually many years. Other organ systems outside the musculoskeletal system may be involved.

Scleroderma (PSS)

Scleroderma is a form of collagen vascular disease. It occurs more commonly in women than men, but not exclusively so. This illness is known by several other terms including "progressive systemic sclerosis" (PSS), and has several subtypes including localized scleroderma called morphia or eosinophylic fasciitis. The illness has several important characteristics, although not entirely unique to PSS, including a characteristic color change of the fingers and hands referred to Raynaud's phenomenon, calcifications just under the skin or calcinosis, diminished esophageal activity which makes swallowing difficult, dilated small blood vessels visible under the skin, especially the face called telangectasia, and tightening of the skin, especially at the fingers called sclerodactyly. Scleroderma literally means "hard skin," and is potentially life-threatening due to damage that occurs to internal organs after excessive accumulation of the protein collagen. Lung or kidney involvement denotes a poor prognosis and encourages aggressive management of complications.

Osteoarthritis (OA)

Degenerative joint disease (DJD) is the most common form of arthritis. Most individuals by age sixty have some evidence of OA. Weight-bearing joints are especially prone to involvement, including the hip, knee, or spine. Modern technology and surgical techniques have made replacements of the hip and knees common, highly successful, and safe in almost every community hospital. Anti-inflammatory medications and mild analgesics provide symptomatic relief, but do not change the course of involvement. Joint trauma results in OA later in life. Whether overuse plays a role in cause remains to be definitely proven. Involvement of the distal interphalangeal joints at the end joint of the finger (Heberden's nodes) and the proximal interphalangeal joint or middle joint of the fingers (Bouchard's joints) affect a unique genetic subset of individuals with OA, usually women. Diffuse idiopathic skeletal hyperostosis (DISH) is a severe form of DJD.

Rheumatoid Arthritis

Rheumatoid arthritis occurs in one percent of the adult American population or greater than two million people. It is clearly more common in women as compared to men, in a ratio of about three to one. It frequently affects people in their most productive years, which is between the ages twenty and forty-five with the peak between thirty-five and forty-five. Disability because of RA results in major economic losses.

> *"Rheumatoid arthritis is an incredibly complex auto-immune disease which results in significant impairment in a patient's quality of life. As our understanding of the immune system grows so will our ability to provide new drugs to treat this devastating disease."*

Leland Loose, Ph.D.
Pfizer Central Research
Groton, Connecticut

Description

Most people affected by RA develop a positive blood test called a rheumatoid factor. Those with a negative blood test or early disease are difficult to diagnose, but have a better prognosis. The fluctuating course characterized by peaks and valleys of activity, or good and bad times, makes it difficult to clearly define the arthritis early. A small number of individuals with new onset RA will have a short-lived illness, which will resolve after a few months. Future research may learn that these people did not have RA or that there are several forms. Most individuals will have a lifetime of disease with development of joint destruction, deformity, and disability. Another small number of patients will have a severe form of the disease referred to as "arthritis mutilans," and never have any periods of inactivity. Recent studies reveal an increase in death rates as compared to the general population, especially in those individuals with severe progressive joint involvement. Those with mul-

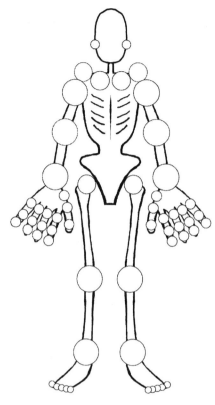

Figure One
The homunculus is a schematic drawing demonstrating the most common joints affected by arthritis. This drawing is an easy way to keep track of painful and swollen joints.

tiple joint involvement or polyarticular disease, persistent swelling, a positive rheumatoid factor in the blood, or evidence by x-ray of bone destruction called erosions have a greater probability of more severe disease than those who do not have these findings. Joint damage and destruction occurs early during the course of the disease.

The arthritis usually affects the hands and feet as compared to the central joints of the body, like the spine. Organ systems outside the musculoskeletal system affected by RA include the skin, blood vessels, eyes, lungs, nervous system, and heart.

Specific joint involvement is characteristic of RA. The examination of the hands by the arthritis specialist is like the chest x-ray is to the lung specialist. At first the hand appears normal, but later changes help define the arthritis.

Joints squeezed during a robust hand shake are painful. Late in the disease the fingers at

CRITERIA FOR THE CLASSIFICATION OF RHEUMATOID ARTHRITIS

- Morning stiffness lasting at least one hour
- Arthritis of 3 or more joints (at least 3 joints simultaneously)
- Arthritis of hand joints (at least one joint swollen)
- Symmetrical joint swelling
- Subcutaneous nodules or lumps under the skin
- X-ray changes of the hands and wrists (erosions)
- A positive blood test for rheumatoid factor

Loss of motion is common at the elbow and results in the inability to fully straighten out the arm or flexion contractures. Flexion at the elbow is preserved, since the hand is brought to the body so many times during the day. Rarely are the hands and arms put out straight from the body during daily activities. It is more difficult to see swelling at the shoulder, but if it does occur it is significant. Holding the shoulder motionless because of pain results in loss of motion and a frozen shoulder called an adhesive capsulitis. Regaining lost shoulder motion is difficult. The loss of motion occurs quickly in a few days,

the largest knuckles of the hands (MCP's) fall down and shift towards the little finger because of the tendons pulling in that direction. Partial dislocation of the last joint of the thumb results in a Z-shaped deformity or 90–90 thumb and makes a good pinch difficult. Swelling over the wrist is common and results in loss of motion. Since a painful joint is often held down or in flexion, grip strength is diminished. Occasionally, swelling over the wrist results in rupture of the tendons, making it impossible to lift up the fourth or fifth fingers. Rheumatoid nodules are common at the elbow and occur in conjunction with swelling of the elbow bursa.

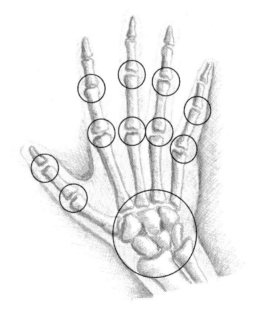

Figure Two
Rheumatoid arthritis primarily affects the joints marked in this drawing.

when a joint is not moved regularly or held motionless.

When the knees are involved, the muscles above the knees shrink and weaken. Quadriceps wasting or weakened quadriceps muscles makes climbing stairs and getting out of a low chair or off the toilet seat difficult. Simple exercises slow this process and improve strength. An elevated toilet seat or seat cushion makes life more tolerable.

Joint fluid accumulates in the back of the knee because of the formation of a "ball and valve" mechanism. This mechanism forms a one-way valve that keeps sending more and more fluid to the back of the knee. The area behind the knee gets tight and tense. A popliteal cyst or Baker's cyst forms that can rupture. If this cyst ruptures it creates a sudden onset of pain and swelling down the calf, oftentimes mimicking deep venous thrombosis. Deep venous thrombosis results in dangerous blood clots in the legs that break off, go

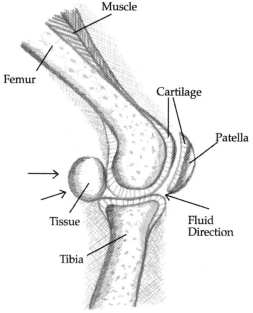

Figure Three

A popliteal cyst forms at the back of the knee when fluid is formed as a consequence of inflammation in the front of the knee. The fluid goes to the back of the knee, but tissue blocks the flow of fluid back to the front. This forms a one-way valve mechanism and fluid accumulates. The area behind the knee gets tight and uncomfortable.

to the lungs, and cause death. Recognizing the difference between these problems is important.

In the foot the toes tend to go in the opposite direction of the fingers, that is, up. This puts extra pressure during weight-bearing on the bottom of the feet over the heads of the bones in that area called metatarsalgia. Calluses form over these same areas. Cocked-up toes rub on shoes and cause skin irritation and sometimes skin ulcers that can get infected. The forefoot widens and deviation of the big toes occur called bunions. A widened forefoot makes it difficult to find shoeware that fits, is comfortable, and doesn't rub on the top of the toes. Involvement of the joint below the ankle causes the foot to sway outward. It looks like you are walking on the side of the foot.

Although the jaw joint, temporal mandibular joint or TMJ joint is often involved, symptoms of locking or pain with chewing don't cause many problems. Individuals don't often realize that there are joints on each side of the vocal cords of the larynx. Inflammation of these joints causes hoarseness or sore throat.

As the disease progresses, hip involvement becomes more likely. Early pain is localized to the groin or even radiates to the knee. Later, hip arthritis results in more widespread or night pain. Limping is common. Use of a cane on the nonpainful side is helpful, and shifts the weight to the other side, but is also difficult if there is arthritis of the hands and wrists too.

Except for the upper cervical spine like the first and second cervical vertebra, most areas of the back and spine are spared by the involvement of RA. A separation of the first two vertebras is common and initially won't cause symptoms. This finding is frequent in those individuals with more severe disease. A modest separation is significant and often requires surgery. At surgery, the two bones are fused together to prevent further separation and any pressure or damage to the spinal cord created by the separated vertebras.

The cause of RA is uncertain. Although not entirely understood, on occasion more than one family member may have RA. Genetic counseling is not necessary, nor is this a reason for those with RA not to have children. Genes that influence the immune system may be inherited and create a susceptibility to the disease. RA is not inherited from parents to children. Unknown factors cause the disease in those individuals with a genetically susceptible immune system. Some researchers believe the unknown factor is an infectious agent that triggers the immune system to react abnormally. RA is not believed to be contagious. Environmental factors play a role. Pregnancy is associated with remissions during the third trimester with subsequent exacerbation in the postpartum period. This suggests hormonal factors play a role in disease activity. Treatment does not rid the body of the cause of the disease, but interrupts the inflammation and destruction of the joint and cartilage.

Destruction of the Joint

A typical joint has a capsule that surrounds the entire joint. The capsule attaches to the bone after the cartilage. This leaves an exposed area of bare bone. The surface inside the capsule is lined by cells usually one or two cell layers thick called synovium. A microscope is necessary to see this in the normal joint. In RA the synovium thickens and develops synovitis when the cells multiply. The synovium is aggressive, invading the exposed area of bare bone just above the normal cartilage. This proliferative synovium becomes so thickened that it is detected by the naked eye. Synovitis really means the same as the term arthritis. If bone destruction

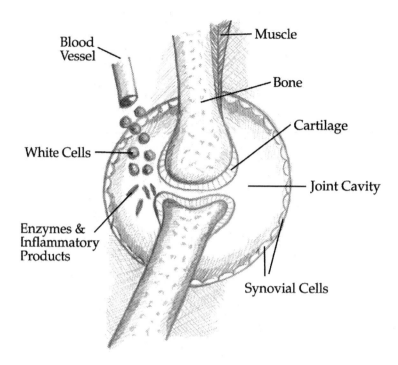

Blood Vessel

Muscle

Bone

Cartilage

White Cells

Enzymes & Inflammatory Products

Joint Cavity

Synovial Cells

Figure Four

This drawing represents a typical joint. The ends of two bones come together. Each end is covered by cartilage. The capsule encloses the entire area and attaches on the bone just above the cartilage. This bare bone is exposed to the joint cavity without protection. The lining of the joint cavity is made up of just few cell layers of synovial cells only seen with the aid of a microscope. Blood vessels, tendons, and muscles are all outside the joint cavity.

occurs around the joint, erosion develops and the joint becomes deformed.

Periarticular erosions or bone destruction around or near the joint is characteristic of RA as compared to the destruction caused by other types of arthritis. You might think the thickened synovium or pannus as it is called would be a good blockade and prevent material from getting into the joint space, but instead, the synovium becomes leaky and allows fluid, cells, and destructive enzymes from the blood stream to enter into the joint. These materials hurt and destroy cartilage, and result in an appearance of melting cartilage or uniform narrowing of the joint space.

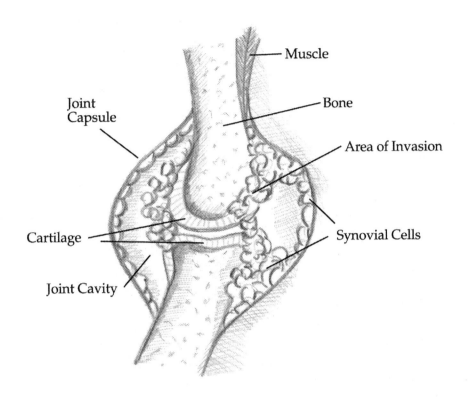

Muscle

Bone

Area of Invasion

Joint Capsule

Cartilage

Joint Cavity

Synovial Cells

Figure Five

This schematic representation of a rheumatoid joint demonstrates an erosion in the bone secondary to the invasion by the synovium cells or lining of the joint cavity. The synovial cells multiply so much they are visible to the naked eye.

Thickened or "turned on" synovium in RA is the most important evidence of the disease. The area around the joint becomes vascular because small blood vessels come into the area. Biopsying the synovium is not a helpful way to make the diagnosis, since it reveals nonspecific inflammation under the microscope. The narrowing of the joint seen on standard x-ray is different than the x-ray changes of osteoarthritis. In OA the joint is narrowed irregularly, not uniformly. The bones adjacent to the joint develop spurs as they form new bone in an attempt of repair in OA. Physicians who read x-rays or radiologists can sort out the differences between various forms of arthritis.

Prognosis

Treatment requires an assessment of prognosis. The prognosis is determined by the history of the natural course and onset of the arthritis, evidence on examination of persistent pain and swelling, laboratory findings, and x-ray evaluations during the first few years of disease. Poor prognosis deserves more aggressive treatment.

Extra-articular involvement of RA or involvement outside the joint and musculoskeletal system significantly affects prognosis and the severity of disease and ultimately treatment. Extra-articular manifestations include a low red blood count or anemia, bumps felt just under the skin especially at the elbows called rheumatoid nodules, a positive blood test marker for RA or rheumatoid factor, and other organ involvement outside the musculoskeletal system. Breathing is compromised when lung involvement oc-

curs. Stiffening of the lung fields referred to as fibrosis, pulmonary nodules that resemble cancer or infection, and fluid accumulation or pleurisy and pleural effusion between the lungs and chest wall all are part of the pulmonary involvement of RA.

DETERMINING THE PROGNOSIS OF RHEUMATOID ARTHRITIS

- Early age at onset
- A positive rheumatoid factor
- An elevated sedimentation rate
- Rheumatoid nodules
- Lung involvement
- Acute inflammation of the eye
- Inflammation of blood vessels
- Inflammation of the heart sack
- Low blood counts and infections

Osteoporosis

Osteoporosis is a loss of the strength of the bones. This condition not only decreases the quality of life, but also adds considerably to the overall cost of health care. Fractures of the spine and hip are major deterrents to a normal quality of life. The related suffering, expense, and inconvenience for patients and family members cannot be measured in a meaningful way. Studies have shown that fifteen to twenty-five percent of elderly women who sustain a fractured hip will lose their independence within the first year after the fracture. The estimated cost of hip fractures in the United States is six to eight billion dollars per year. If the incidence of such fractures could be decreased, the cost savings to society would be substantial.

"Osteoporosis is an illness that until the last few years has been considered an almost inevitable consequence of age. We have known of the terrible consequences to those who have developed

this condition, deformity, severe physical limitations in movement and function, and even death. With an understanding that this illness can be treated and the risks of complications avoided there is hope that another of the serious illnesses that have affected men and women can be conquered. The present need is for patients to seek early diagnosis and treatment and for physicians to make these tests and treatments available."

H. Walter Emori, M.D.
Osteoporosis Center
Medford, Oregon

Description

Osteoporosis simply means having too little density in the bones. This leads to weak, fragile bones, and fractures. The bone becomes more porous. After the mid-thirties, bone loss becomes continuous as a part of the aging process. The greatest bone density achieved is the peak bone mass. This occurs at different ages, but is usually achieved by age thirty. As the bone density diminishes, it falls below a fracture threshold, the level of bone density at which time bone fractures occur much more readily. This occurs from bone loss or developing less peak bone mass initially.

Osteoporosis is a common disease. It is estimated that more than fifty percent of post-menopausal women will be affected. In women, the incidence of osteoporosis is greater than heart attack, breast cancer, and stroke combined. More than one million individuals in America suffer osteoporotic fractures each year. During a woman's lifetime, she will lose an average of thirty to fifty percent of her body's bone density. Four in ten women older than fifty years of age are likely to suffer an osteoporosis-related fracture of the hip, spine, or wrist at some point during the remainder of their lifetimes.

Minor falls or fragility falls are from standing height and can cause fractures of the wrist, hip, spine, or pelvis in those individuals with osteoporosis. Repeated spinal fractures result in the compression of vertebral bodies and reduced height. Repeated fractures result in a dowager's hump or widow's hump, an extreme curvature, kyphosis, and deformity of the upper thoracic spine. This results in loss of height of several inches, difficulty with clothes fitting normally, and pain.

A family history of osteoporosis increases one's risk of osteoporosis. There is a greater risk with low body weight, low dietary calcium intake, excess alcohol, and high caffeine consumption. If you are a nonblack woman your chance of developing osteoporosis during your lifetime is about twenty-five percent. This risk can be cut in half if you begin estrogen replacement therapy as soon as your menstrual cycle stops. A variety of medical treatments promote bone loss, including systemic steroids or anticonvulsant therapy. Early menopause, either naturally or as a result of surgery or oophorectomy, results in bone loss. Immediate estrogen replacement therapy can help. Other medical conditions like kidney disease, endocrine disease, excess thyroid hormone replacement, the loss of menses in young women, and men with a lack of normal male hormone levels may develop osteoporosis. Rarer and less common illnesses are also associated with osteoporosis. Bone loss is usually most rapid during the first few years after menopause and then continues slowly with age.

There is a direct relationship between the density and strength of your bones and the risk for fracture. A bone density test can determine risk for fracture. Dual energy x-ray absorbtiometry or DEXA is a fast, simple, convenient means to determine the bone density measurement or BMD. It is painless and can be done without undressing. Insurance companies recognize and reimburse for bone density measurements. Bone density testing can detect a low bone density before a fracture occurs, predict the chance of a fracture in the future, confirm the diagnosis of osteoporosis, determine the rate of bone loss, and monitor the effects of treatment if the test is conducted at periodic intervals.

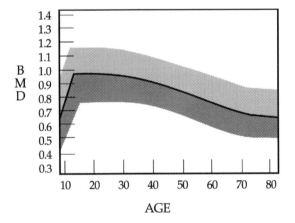

Figure Six
The DEXA report is the most precise and accurate mechanism to measure bone density and the risk for fracture. This is a portion of a typical report.

Treatment
Available medical treatment includes medications that increase bone density.

- *Estrogen replacement therapy* at the time of menopause can positively impact bone loss and is one of the most effective means of preventing fracture from osteoporosis.

- *Calcium* in the amount of 1000 to 1500 mg of calcium replacement a day supplements diets low in calcium. The best natural sources of calcium are dairy products, including whole or skim milk and cheese. Leafy green vegetables, including broccoli, collards, turnip greens, mustard greens, and spinach are also good sources. Salmon, sardines, and raw oysters are high in calcium too. The Recommended Daily Allowance or U.S. RDA of calcium for women age nineteen and over is 1000 mg. Experts feel this is not enough, and recommend 1000 mg a day for women before menopause and as much as 1500 mg daily after menopause to reduce the risk of osteoporosis. It is important to consult your physician before taking large amounts of calcium. Most women get about 500 to 600 mg calcium per day in their diet. This adds to the risk for osteoporosis. For these reasons many women should consider adding calcium tablets to their daily routine. Very high consumption of calcium can increase the risk for kidney stones, especially in those individuals with a prior history. However, less than 2,000 mg daily constitutes a very small risk.

- *Bisphosphonates* are a group of compounds that decrease the loss of bone associated with accelerated or normal bone remodeling. Alendronate (Fosamax) and risedronate (Actonel) are poorly absorbed and must be taken first thing in the morning without any food or other medicines for a minimum of one half hour after it is ingested. Bisphosphonates have been associated with irritation of the esophagus or esophagitis. It is recommended alendronate and risedronate be given after awakening in the morning in an upright position, out of bed, with a full glass of water to minimize irritation. In this way it is well tolerated. An occasional patient may experience some bone pain, aggravation of arthritic complaints, and abdominal pain that will usually resolve on its own.

- *Calcitonin* is given as a subcutaneous injection or nasal spray (Miacalcin). This naturally occurring hormone blocks bone resorption and has been useful in relieving the pain of acute vertebral compression fractures. One spray is directed into the nostril once a day.

- *Raloxifene (Evista)* is a nontraditional hormone. It has been approved by the FDA for use in the prevention of osteoporosis. It is a selective estrogen receptor modulator or SERM. These nontraditional hormones are called "designer estrogens." Raloxifene acts like estrogen in certain tissues, but not in others. Raloxifene can build bone, though not quite as much as estrogen replacements. The effects on decreasing fractures has been beneficial. Because raloxifene acts selectively, most women do not experience bleeding, bloating, and breast tenderness associated with estrogen replacements. Women do not experience an increase of breast cancer or endometrial cancer. Endometrial cancer is cancer of the lining of the uterus. Raloxifene can help lower the blood cholesterol too. This drug will not help the symptoms of hot flashes, insomnia, mood swings, or night sweats, and in some women may precipitate hot flashes. Raloxifene increases the risk of blood clot, and should be discontinued during prolonged periods of immobilization.

- *Vitamin D* in the body is to promote the process of bone mineralization. While calcium and other minerals are the building blocks of healthy bones, it is vitamin D that regulates their actions in the body and makes them available for absorption into bone. Vitamin D can be produced in the body with the help of sunlight. Vitamin D is easily obtained from our diet as well from sunlight. Milk and margarine are fortified with vitamin D as well as many other foods. It occurs naturally in significant amounts in eggs, liver, and fish. Adequate amounts should be consumed daily, but not necessarily at the same time of calcium. Vitamin D needs to be present in the diet on a regular basis along with calcium to perform its functions in the body. The recommended daily allowance

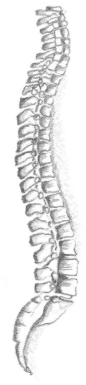

Figure Seven
The spine is a complicated structure made up of a series of bones stacked up on each other in an overlapping manner.

(RDA) of vitamin D is 400 international units (IU). The amount of vitamin D in the diet is well within the recommended limits. Concentrated forms or supplements can result in vitamin D toxicity.

- *Diuretics* minimize the loss of calcium in the urine and are helpful in some people. Other treatments under investigation include powerful forms of vitamin D, newer forms of sodium fluoride, low dose parathyroid hormone, and antiestrogen drugs.

- *Kyphoplasty* is the surgical treatment of vertebral body compression fractures. This procedure is minimally invasive and can relieve the back pain of acute spinal fractures. The procedure can be done in the hospital or as an outpatient while asleep (under general anesthesia) or awake (using local anesthesia). Under the guidance of x-ray, a small tube is placed into the area of the broken bone. This provides a path for the insertion later of a special balloon. When inflated the balloon raises the collapsed bone fractures and creates a space inside the vertebral body. The balloon is then removed and the space filled with material to support the bone. Filling the space prevents further collapse of the vertebral fracture and provides pain relief. Vertebroplasty is a similar procedure, but doesn't utilize the balloon.

The key to the management of osteoporosis is not treatment, but prevention. Regular exercise reduces the risk of fractures by preventing both osteoporosis and falls. Exercise improves gait, balance, coordination and muscle strength. Exercise should be part of the strategy for all individuals with osteoporosis.

Smoking is discouraged!

Systemic Lupus Erythematosus

Systemic Lupus Erythematosus (SLE) is a chronic autoimmune disease that results in inflammation of several areas of the body, especially the skin, joints, blood and kidneys. It is the inflammation of tissues that results in the symptoms of SLE. The illness affects young women of childbearing years, between fifteen to thirty-five years of age. However, the elderly or young are not excluded either. The ratio of women to men is nine to one, that is, nine women get the disease for every one man that gets the disease. Although SLE occurs within families, there is no known gene or genes that are thought to cause the illness. A small percent of lupus patients will have a close relative that already has or may develop lupus. An even smaller percentage of the children born to individuals with lupus will develop the illness. When it comes to lupus, the greatest relationship appears to be mother and daughter. Lupus is often called a "woman's disease," despite the fact that many men are affected. The symptoms of the disease are the same in men and women. People of African, American Indian, and Asian origin are thought to develop the disease more frequently than Caucasian women.

> *"Lupus is a disease with many different spectra. Rare cases are severe and life-threatening, while most are manageable. Many persons who think they have a form of lupus do not, so it is essential that a correct diagnosis be made and toxic therapy not be used. In contrast, patients with severe and active lupus need close management by experienced rheumatologists working closely with primary care physicians."*

Edward D. Harris, Jr., M.D.
Division of Rheumatology
Stanford University School of Medicine
Stanford, California

Hormonal factors may explain why lupus occurs more frequently in females than in males. The increase of disease symptoms before menstrual periods and/or during pregnancy supports the belief that hormones, particularly estrogen, may be involved. However, the exact hormonal reason for the greater prevalence of lupus in women, and the cyclic increase in symptoms is unknown. This is not a reason for lupus patients to avoid birth control pills or estrogen replace-ment therapy during postmenopausal years; however, you should check with your doctor.

The Immune Response

The body's immune system normally makes proteins called antibodies to protect the body against viruses, bacteria, and other foreign materials. These foreign materials are called antigens. In an autoimmune disorder such as lupus, the immune system loses its ability to tell the difference between foreign substances called antigens and its own cells and tissues called "self." The immune system then makes antibodies directed against "self." These antibodies are called "auto-antibodies" and react with the "self" antigens to form immune complexes. The immune complexes deposit in various tissues and create inflammation, injury to tissues, and pain. Over seventy percent of people with lupus have systemic lupus. These antibodies deposit in several different parts of the body. About one half of people with lupus deposit antibodies that damage internal organs and one half of them deposit antibodies outside the internal organs.

Clinical Course of Lupus

More people have lupus than better-recognized diseases like AIDS, cerebral palsy, multiple sclerosis, sickle-cell anemia and cystic fibrosis combined. A number of other diseases are closely related, or may be part of the same disease including mixed connective tissue disease (MCTD), scleroderma or progressive systemic sclerosis (PSS), polymyositis (PM) or dermatomyositis (DM), rheumatoid arthritis (RA), and Sjögren's syndrome (SS).

About five percent of lupus patients have overlap syndromes or a combination of symptoms. For the most part, lupus is a mild disease affecting only a few organs, but it may cause serious and even life-threatening problems. It is helpful to think of the disease as a long railroad track or ladder, with the more serious manifestations of the disease like kidney inflammation (nephritis) or brain inflammation (cerebritis) at one end, and minor symptoms like rash or joint pain at the other end. Joint pain or arthralgia without actual swelling of joints is a prominent part of the disease. There are a number of people that seem to have one foot on the track and the other on shaky ground. These individuals cannot definitely be diagnosed, but have an ill-defined connective disease that may blossom to lupus in the future. The close monitoring of these individuals is important. The disease is characterized by remissions and exacerbations, good times or bad times called flares, so that individuals can move up and down the track in either direction. This occurs over weeks, months, or years.

Criteria for the Diagnosis

Although lupus can affect any organ system of the body, most people experience symp-toms in only a few organs. Many of the symptoms mimic other illnesses and are sometimes vague. Because the disease course is characterized by remissions and exacerbations, lupus can be difficult to diagnose. The diagnosis is made by a careful review of an individual's medical history, an analysis of the results obtained in routine laboratory tests, and specialized tests related to the patient's immune status.

Currently, there is no single laboratory test that can determine whether a person has lupus.

The antinuclear antibody, or ANA, is a marker for disease, but it must be put in perspective. It is widely accepted as a screening test. Some have suggested the disease is on the increase, however, there is more likely a greater awareness of lupus. The utilization of the ANA blood test in combination with awareness of the disease and its symptoms has resulted in an easier diagnosis. The ANA is positive in virtually all people with systemic lupus and is the best diagnostic test for systemic lupus available. If the test is negative, the patient most likely does not have systemic lupus erythematosus.

The American College of Rheumatology (ACR) has provided a list of eleven symptoms or signs that help distinguish lupus from other diseases. A person should have four or more of these criteria to suspect lu-

THE ELEVEN CRITERIA FOR THE DIAGNOSIS OF LUPUS

Malar Rash

- A rash over the cheeks and bridge of the nose in a butterfly distribution

Discoid Rash

- Scaly red raised patches commonly on the face and neck

Photosensitivity

- Reaction to sunlight and an increase in skin rash

Oral Ulcers

- Sores in the nose or mouth, usually painless

Arthritis

- Arthritis in at least two joints in which the bones around the joints do not become destroyed or deformed

Serositis

- Inflammation of the lining around the heart, lungs, or abdomen

Kidney

- Excessive protein in the urine and/or elements derived from red or white cells or kidney cells

Neurologic

- Seizures, convulsions, or psychosis in the absence of drugs or disturbances that are known to cause such effects

Blood

- Hemolytic anemia or the rupture of red blood cells, leukopenia or low white cells, or thrombocytopenia or low platelets
- Platelets plug up holes in the blood stream and prevent bleeding

Immunologic

- A positive anti-DNA test or specific autoantibody for SLE, positive anti-Sm test, false positive syphilis test (VDRL) or evidence of the antiphospholipid syndrome on the blood tests

Antibody

- A positive test for antinuclear antibodies (ANA) in the absence of drugs known to induce it pus. The symptoms do not all have to occur at the same time.

A positive ANA, by itself, is not diagnostic of lupus, since the test is also positive in other conditions.

CONDITIONS ASSOCIATED WITH POSITIVE ANAS

- Other connective tissue disorders
- Older individuals; the elderly
- Secondary to certain drugs
- Inflammatory conditions that are chronic, like infectious mononucleosis and other infections, leprosy, subacute bacterial endocarditis, malaria, and liver disease

---

The ANA test is reported as either positive or negative. If positive, the results include a titer. The titer indicates how many times an individual's blood must be diluted to get a sample free of antinuclear antibodies. Typically, the laboratory begins with testing 1:20, then 1:40, 1:80, 1:160, 1:320, 1:640, 1:1280 and so on. A titer of 1:640 has greater concentration of antinuclear antibodies than a titer of 1:320 or 1:160. The test does not determine activity of disease and should be utilized for a marker of disease only, rather than determining the need for therapy. The higher titers do have importance, however.

Patients with active lupus have ANA tests that are very high in titer. Laboratory tests that measure complement levels in the blood are also of some value. Complement is a circulating blood protein that destroys bacteria with antibodies. It is an "amplifier" of the immune system. If the total blood complement level is low, it suggests that antigen-antibody complexes combined with complement are being deposited in the tissues and the lupus is active. Other markers of disease include the anti-DNA antibody, the anti-Sm antibody, the anti-RNP antibody, and the anti-Ro antibody. The anti-DNA correlates to activity of disease and is helpful in determining the need for treatment. Some antibodies are specific to lupus, activity of disease, or unique problems occurring in lupus patients. Skin biopsies of both a lupus rash and normal skin help diagnose systemic lupus. The interpretation of these tests is frequently difficult.

The most common blood abnormality in lupus is anemia; a reduction in the number of red blood cells (RBCs) in the circulation. About one half of the patients are anemic. This results in fatigue. There are several reasons for the lupus patient to be anemic, including impaired kidney function, bleeding, inflammation at the site of red blood cell production in the bone marrow, and the premature destruction of red blood cells as a result of antibodies directed against red blood cells in the circulation. In patients with kidney failure, an injectable red-cell-stimulating hormone, erythropoietin (Epogen), helps stimulate the production of red blood cells.

The platelets are tiny circulating particles in the blood that prevent bleeding by plugging areas of leakage in the circulation. A deficiency of these elements called thrombocytopenia, results in excessive bruising of the skin or bleeding. This bleeding tendency is aggravated by the use of aspirin, since aspirin thins the blood by making the platelets less sticky and less effective in plugging leaks. This aspirin effect lasts the lifetime of platelets, usually several days after aspirin is stopped. NSAIDs have the same effect on the platelets, but only while they are being taken. The COX-2 anti-inflammatories do not have an effect on platelets. A bone marrow biopsy examines where the platelets are formed and determines whether the deficiency is a result of destruction in the circulation or diminished production. Increased destruction is benefited by the removal of the spleen or splenectomy. Newer technologies and surgical skills allow this organ to be removed safely through a scope put through the abdominal wall. Other antibodies in the circulation include the lupus anticoagulant. This antibody results in clotting rather than bleeding. This requires treatment with blood thinners like heparin by injection or oral coumadin. Finally, the white blood cells may be reduced (leukopenia) in lupus, and if severe, there is an increased susceptibility to infection. Sometimes unusual infections called "opportunistic infections" occur. Some lupus patients require prophylactic antibiotics or a white cell stimulating drug, Neupogen. Vaccinations to prevent infection are encouraged. Patients having a splenectomy should always have a pneumococcal vaccination before the spleen is removed, since these patients are at risk for increased pneumococcal infections.

Lupus nephritis is the term used most often to describe the inflammation of the kidney as a result of this disease.

It is estimated that about one third of patients with lupus will develop nephritis requiring medical evaluation and treatment.

This is a potentially serious aspect of lupus. There are few signs or symptoms and the course of nephritis is highly variable. Often the only abnormality is discovered in the urine analysis. This is usually mild, however, the lupus patient with more serious involvement has the potential to lose kidney function. The loss of protein through the kidney (nephrotic syndrome) results in fluid retention, weight gain, and edema or ankle swelling. A kidney biopsy helps determine the prognosis and necessary treatment. Despite treatment, some patients with lupus still go on to develop kidney failure. This requires artificial hemodialysis or peritoneal dialysis at home. Dialysis cleans the blood artificially. Kidney transplantation has been successful in those patients with loss of complete kidney function, and eliminates the need for long-term dialysis. Lupus patients may develop kidney infections or hypertension. NSAIDs aggravate the deterioration of kidney function. These problems are treated with appropriate medication.

Treatment of Lupus

Preventive measures reduce the risk of flares. For photosensitive patients, avoidance of excessive sun exposure and the regular application of sunscreens will usually prevent rashes. Regular exercise helps prevent muscle weakness and fatigue. Immunization protects against specific infections. Estrogen replacement, weight-bearing exercise, calcium and vitamin D supplements during menopause preserve bone density, minimizing osteoporosis and the risk for bone fracture. Support groups help alleviate the effects of stress. Treatment approaches are based on the symptoms.

For the vast majority of people with lupus, effective treatment can minimize symptoms, reduce inflammation, and maintain normal functions.

The course of lupus varies among people. Medications are prescribed for people with lupus depending on which organs are involved, and the severity of involvement.

Drug-induced lupus occurs after the use of certain prescribed drugs in a small number of people—only a few percent. The symp-toms of drug-induced lupus are similar to those of systemic lupus. A large percentage of patients who take these drugs will develop antibodies suggestive of lupus; of those only a small number will develop actual drug-induced lupus. The symptoms usually resolve when the medications are discontinued.

Pregnancy and Lupus

A concern for many families is whether a young woman with lupus should risk becoming pregnant. Pregnancy poses unique and special problems for women with lupus. Even so, there is no reason why a woman with lupus should not get pregnant. Other organ involvement like the central nervous system, kidney, or heart and lungs that are currently active, would place the mother at risk. There is some increased risk of disease activity during or immediately after pregnancy. If a person is monitored carefully, the danger can be minimized.

A pregnant woman with lupus should be followed closely by both her obstetrician and rheumatologist during her pregnancy.

Another problem with lupus patients is the antiphospholipid syndrome. Antiphospholipid antibodies are responsible for many of the problems a pregnant lupus patient has carrying a fetus to full term. Pregnant women with lupus have more stillbirths, premature deliveries, smaller birth weights, and miscarriages than individuals without lupus. On occasion babies of mothers with lupus receive

COMMONLY PRESCRIBED MEDICATIONS FOR LUPUS PATIENTS

Nonsteroidal Anti-Inflammatory Drugs (NSAIDs)

• Recommended for muscle pain, joint pain, or arthritis.

Acetaminophen

• A mild analgesic that is used for pain. It has the advantage of less stomach irritation than aspirin, but it is not nearly as effective at suppressing inflammation.

Corticosteroids or steroids

• Hormones that have anti-inflammatory and immunoregulatory properties. Synthetically produced steroids are used to reduce inflammation and suppress the activity of the immune system. The most commonly prescribed steroid drug is prednisone. Steroids have a variety of side effects, so the dose must be closely monitored.

Antimalarials

• Antimalarials are used to treat malaria, but are also useful in the treatment of lupus. There is no known relationship between lupus and malaria. Antimalarials are useful in the skin and joint symptoms of lupus, and have few side effects. The effect takes several weeks to occur. Eye toxicity rarely occurs, but can be detected by regular and early eye exams.

Cytotoxics

• These drugs kill cells that are rapidly dividing and suppress the immune system. They can predispose to cancer and infection. Regular laboratory monitoring is necessary. Early treatment may reduce complications of disease and diminish the time necessary for these medications.

Sunscreen

• Sun protection factor (SPF) of fifteen or more helps block exposure to the sun. The majority of lupus patients are sensitive to sun exposure, and for some exposure can result in generalized flares with symptoms of fever, joint pain, or more systemic involvement. Sun exposure can be prevented by wearing hats with a brim, long-sleeved shirts, and other clothing to protect from direct sun exposure. Total avoidance of the sun for most people is not necessary.

antibodies that cross the placenta from the mother to the baby. These antibodies (Ro antibodies) cause heart blockage for the baby at the time of birth. Often this can be anticipated and planned interventions can be ready at birth. The heart blockage is usually transient.

If a lupus patient plans or anticipates pregnancy, it is important that the disease is fairly quiescent and there is little need for medicine.

Pregnancy does not need to be totally avoided. Many lupus patients have healthy children and large families.

Antimalarials are fetal toxic and should not be utilized during pregnancy. Steroids in low doses can be used safely during pregnancy. If the doctor advises against pregnancy or children are not wanted, it is important to practice effective birth control measures. Even though fertility is decreased, unplanned pregnancy can occur. The safest form of birth control for women with lupus is a diaphragm with contraceptive foam, but birth controls pills may be used safely most of the time.

Discoid Lupus

Discoid lupus is a variant of lupus and is limited to the skin. It occurs in about ten percent of people with lupus. It is identified by a characteristic rash that appears on the face, neck, and scalp. The diagnosis is made by examining a biopsy of the rash. Discoid lupus does not involve the body's internal organs. It is not systemic. The antinuclear antibody may be negative in patients with discoid lupus. In a large number of patients with discoid lupus the ANA test is positive, but at a low level. A small percentage of discoid lupus patients will evolve into the systemic form of the disease. This cannot be predicted or prevented.

Treatment of discoid lupus will not prevent its progression to the systemic form. Individuals who progress to the systemic form probably had systemic lupus at the outset, with the discoid rash as their main symptom complex. Systemic lupus is usually more severe than discoid lupus and can affect almost any organ or system of the body. Lupus presents itself differently in every individual. It is difficult to make comparisons from one person's illness to another. When people mention "lupus," they are usually referring to the systemic form of the disease.

Mixed Connective Tissue Disease

Mixed connective tissue disease (MCTD) was originally described as a syndrome that consisted of a combination of features typically found in patients with systemic lupus erythematosus, systemic sclerosis, polymyositis/dermatomyositis, or rheumatoid arthritis. The blood test that differentiates MCTD from other connective tissue diseases is a positive ANA in a speckled pattern (under a special microscope) and the presence of other autoantibodies, RNP. MCTD as a distinct entity has been a matter of controversy. Some of the patients with MCTD develop clinical symptoms compatible with the presence of a well-defined CTD. Originally, MCTD was defined as a relatively benign disorder, but now has been associated with significant organ involvement similar to other serious CTDs. Finally, the autoantibody first described in MCTD has now also been seen in other CTDs. These reasons have led some experts to suggest MCTD be referred to as "undifferentiated" CTD, or an "overlap" syndrome.

Prognosis of Lupus

The idea that lupus is generally a fatal disease is a misconception. The prognosis of lupus is much better today than ever before. With early diagnosis, new and changing methods of therapy—including the judicious use of medications—80 to 90 percent of people with lupus can look forward to a normal life span. Prior to current medical advances most patient deaths were the result of kidney failure or involvement of the central nervous system. Today, as many patients with lupus will die from infection as from active disease. Lupus patients are more susceptible to infection because of the effects of the disease on their immune status. These effects reduce their ability to prevent or fight infection. Many of the medications suppress the immune response, leaving the patient more prone to infection also. Although some people with lupus have severe recurrent attacks and are frequently hospitalized, most people with lupus rarely require hospitalization. There are many lupus patients who never have to be hospitalized. The course remains unpredictable.

It is therefore a sensible idea to maintain control of a disease that tomorrow may be curable!

Fibromyalgia

Fibromyalgia is an increasingly recognized disorder. It is also known as soft-tissue rheumatism, fibrositis, or nonarticular rheumatism. Some people call it a myofascial pain syndrome. It is characterized by widespread aches and pains, associated fatigue, and poor sleep. It is one of the most common problems for which people seek the advice of a physician. It is believed that two percent of the American population has fibromyalgia. Arthritis sufferers may also have fibromyalgia, yet fibromyalgia is really not a form of arthritis and will not harm the joints. A wealth of information has been written about fibromyalgia.

"As a general internist, I often see patients with multiple complaints, both physical and psychological. After ruling out other diagnostic possibilities, fibromyalgia must be considered. Acknowledgment of this diagnosis and persis-

tence with the various treatment options will often result in significant reduction in pain and improvement in patient's sense of well-being."

Ron Smith, M.D., Ph.D.
Internal Medicine
Reno, Nevada

It appears that there are at least three important aspects with regard to this illness. There is some element of sleep disturbance. Individuals don't get deep sleep or stage four sleep. They toss and turn. They are "fitful sleepers." They get up at night with pain or discomfort, and rather than fall back asleep quickly, they actually stay awake or get out of bed. Upon wakening they are not rested. Later, during the day, they have difficulty coping with other problems. Sleep disturbance need not be the first symptom, but occurs in conjunction with the other symptoms of fibromyalgia.

Fibromyalgia has long been linked to psychological disturbance. The patients are depressed, discouraged, or distressed. They don't always see the "light at the end of the tunnel." They are fatigued and lack energy or endurance.

Characteristic tender points have been well mapped out. Trigger points occur at the base of the skull, neck and shoulders, elbows, low back, breast bone, hips, or the knees. These areas are extremely painful to touch. The pain is very real. If you take a scalpel and cut across these areas, nothing is found, even under the microscope. When touched or palpated, the response in these areas is usually abrupt withdrawal, out of proportion to the pressure applied. You may not be aware of these areas until examined.

This syndrome is a collection of symptoms without a definite test to define it. It quickly becomes a vicious cycle. The cycle easily escalates and snowballs. There may be a precipitating event, like a back injury, car accident, or fall. Fibromyalgia can be disabling. If symptoms occur for a short while, the prognosis is much better than symptoms ongoing for a long period of time. At the time of diagnosis, most people have had many years of symptoms.

There is no routine laboratory test or x-ray procedure that is of diagnostic or of prognostic value in fibromyalgia.

Criteria
The American College of Rheumatology established criteria to identify the syndrome. These criteria appear to be relatively simple, sensitive, and specific. Some critics suggest that individuals should not be mislabeled with this diagnosis; however, many people are subjected to unnecessary diagnostic tests

and in some cases surgery before the diagnosis is well established. Establishing the label early may in fact prevent unnecessary testing and procedures. The pain precipitates a withdrawal response from the patient.

CRITERIA TO ESTABLISH FIBROMYALGIA

- Widespread pain for three months on both right and left sides of the body
- Pressure applied to at least eleven out of eighteen trigger points

---

Treatment

Surgery should be avoided and narcotics kept to a minimum. The lack of understanding the basis of the disease results in the therapy being empiric. Pain cannot be cut out. Unfortunately, many of these individuals have been subjected to surgeries in an attempt to rid them of pain.

If you operate for only pain, you get more pain.

Narcotics do not get at the source of the problem. Many times narcotics provide an opportunity for abuse, dependence, and even addiction. Early treatment should be non-pharmacological, and include counseling, exercise, and education. When these methods fail, antidepressant medications at night

or muscle relaxants are helpful. Many medications help with the sleep disturbance, improve mood eventually, and elevate the brain's threshold for pain without creating dependency. Interventions that break the vicious cycle of pain, poor sleep, and depression will be of benefit. Local steroid injections, massage, or physical therapy are helpful and have little risk. Individuals may seek alternative treatment providers including the chiropractor, massage therapist, or acupuncturist. All will be helpful to some degree.

Treatment should always be conservative.

Tricyclic antidepressants like amitriptyline (Elavil) and muscle relaxants like cyclobenzaprine (Flexeril) appear to be effective in the short-term treatment of fibromyalgia and have been available in the United States for over thirty years. With these agents most people will have a modest degree of improvement. Some will have dramatic improvement of symptoms. It is impossible to identify who will respond. Since the side effects of these medicines are mild and resolve quickly with discontinuation of medication, treatment is warranted. Amitriptyline in low doses should be the initial medication. The dose should be taken at bedtime to help the sleep disturbance, and earlier in the evening if there is morning-after sedation. Early side effects like dry mouth or excessive sedation will improve with time. Medication may be continued for several months and then tapered or discontinued. In some situations medicine is continued for years. Other common side effects of tricyclic antidepressants include weight gain, nightmares, constipation, dreaming, and occasional paradoxical insomnia. These medications are relatively inexpensive.

It is unclear whether antidepressants that are selective serotonin reuptake inhibitors (SSRIs) like Prozac, Paxil, or Zoloft are of more value than traditional tricyclic antidepressants. More people discontinue treatment with tricyclic antidepressants because of side effects, than do people taking SSRIs. Antianxiety medications are of limited value. Early enthusiasm for them has been tempered by the concern for dependence and possible withdrawal symptoms. Anti-inflammatory medications, except for their mild effect on pain appear to have little if any value in the treatment of fibromyalgia.

Individuals with fibromyalgia often fall prey to unproven remedies or unconventional treatment programs. Although these may not do any harm, they raise false hope. You are then crushed or broken-hearted when there is no relief. Unproven remedies lighten the pocketbook, since most are relatively expensive.

Local injection of tender points with steroids and anesthetic are utilized with some success. Injections should be limited in number. Chiropractic manipulation and myofascial therapy like "spray and stretch" have also had limited success. Education and exercise are important ingredients and adjuvants of any treatment program for the fibromyalgia patient.

Fibromyalgia should not be interpreted as a disabling or crippling condition, but rather as a chronic disorder with available effective therapies. There is no cure. Patients must take an active role in their treatment as compared to a passive role. Patient support groups are helpful.

The role of victim must be discouraged!

Fibromyalgia is a disorder of exclusion. It is important to ensure that other illnesses that could explain the symptoms are not present. Hypothyroidism or other more serious disease could be confused with the symptoms of fibromyalgia. It occurs more frequently with other rheumatic illnesses including rheumatoid arthritis. Other serious illnesses can be associated with mood changes, poor sleep, and pain. An examination by a medical doctor can sort out these other problems.

There may be an overlap between fibromyalgia and chronic fatigue syndrome. Similarities suggest that these two syndromes are possibly the same thing at different ends of the same spectrum of disease.

Gout

Gout is one of the best examples of acute or inflammatory arthritis. Crystals of uric acid create a sudden inflammatory response by the body. In the joint the crystal creates acute swelling, redness, warmth, and pain. Uric acid concentrations fluctuate. During an acute attack of gout, the uric acid concentration may not be elevated, since the levels can fluctuate.

> "Gout is a form of arthritis originally referred to as the 'disease of kings.' The first descriptions date back to the days of Babylon. We now understand the cause of the disease. Prevention is possible through the use of medications. I wish this could be said about other rheumatic diseases as well."

Teresa Bachman, M.D.
Rheumatologist
Reno, Nevada

Uric acid concentrations should be monitored over several weeks to determine if they are elevated, not only at the time of an attack. Fluctuations up or down are often responsible for precipitating an acute attack. A low uric measurement does not exclude the diagnosis of gout.

The blood uric acid level is still the most important determinant of the risk for developing gout.

Description

The first attack of gout involves one big toe over fifty percent of the time. It is referred to as podagra. Ninety-five percent of the time during the course of gouty arthritis, an attack will occur in the big toe. The first attack may occur in other lower extremity joints including the knee, ankle, or foot. An acute attack occurring in several joints at the same time is polyarticular gout. Men get their first attack of gout in about the third decade of life, unless there is a rare inherited problem with metabolism. Women get gout after menopause. Gout is an unusual occurrence in the young. Gout is recognized as the most common form of acute arthritis in males over forty years of age.

It is not unusual to go to bed fine and wake up with a severely swollen, red, and painful big toe in the morning.

Without intervention, gout is a self-limiting condition; it will resolve on its own. Unfortunately, until it does, the person is miserable. For that reason, individuals seek out urgent medical attention. The inflammation is acute and can be associated with systemic conditions, even fever. The inflammation mimics infection. Treatment to suppress the inflammation is very different from decreasing the uric acid levels. Untreated gout lasts several days. Until it resolves, the discomfort is severe. Gout is often frequent and recurrent. Treatment results in relief in a matter of hours with complete resolution in a few days.

Treatment

An acute attack requires a different drug treatment than the underlying hyperuricemia condition. During an acute attack, the treatment is directed against the inflammation. Nonsteroidal anti-inflammatories (NSAIDs) are helpful and should be started at the first sign of an attack. Patients with recurrent gout usually recognize signs and symptoms early and often abort full-blown gout attacks with medicine. Indomethacin (Indocin/Indocin SR) has been a favorite NSAID, but most all NSAIDs are helpful including the selective COX-2 agents. High doses of NSAIDs early, followed by tapering doses can bring rapid relief. On occasion, it is necessary to use oral steroids or even intra-articular steroids. Infection must be ruled out. Steroids by either route work quite well and quickly. The drug colchicine has also been used for many years in acute attacks of gout. Colchicine is one of the oldest remedies for gout. There are three indications for the use of colchicine in the treatment of gout. The control of acute gouty arthritis, colchicine prophylaxis for the treatment of interval gout, and the prophylactic colchicine administration during initial therapy with allopurinol or drugs that encourage the excretion of uric acid into the urine. Once considered the mainstay in the treatment of acute gout, colchicine is now used infrequently because of its adverse effects. Colchicine is more effective when used early, especially during the first twenty-four hours of onset of an acute gouty attack. All too often patients do not start taking it until a day or so following the onset of an attack. Oral colchicine is useful in two-thirds of patients presenting with acute gout. Many people however, experience nausea, vomiting, diarrhea, and abdominal pain before full improvement. This narrow benefit to toxicity ratio has limited the use of colchicine. NSAIDs are generally better tolerated, more efficacious, and are the first choice of most rheumatologists in the treatment of acute gouty arthritis. The pill is so small it looks like a bird seed.

The underlying problem in gout is an elevated uric acid. Either too much uric acid is produced by the body or too little is excreted by the kidneys. It is common to treat elevated uric acid concentrations with the drug allopurinol (Zyloprim), which inhibits the production of uric acid, or the drug probenecid (Benemid), which increases the excretion of uric acid in the urine. Increasing the amount of uric acid in the urine is not desirable if kidney stones have been a problem. Elevated uric acid concentrations lead to more frequent gout attacks and more severe attacks. Eventually, the attacks occur more often and are more painful.

Gout occurs in three overlapping stages that include a long phase of asymptomatic elevated uric acid levels called hyperuricemia, a period of recurrent acute gouty attacks of sudden onset, separated by asymptomatic intervals or periods without symptoms, followed in about ten percent of patients by chronic tophaceous gouty arthritis. Tophi are large collections of uric acid crystals deposited in the connective tissues outside the joints. Tophi are common in patients with untreated or inadequately treated elevated uric acid levels. Gout is one of the better-understood rheumatic diseases and certainly one of the most gratifying to treat.

Prevention of gouty arthritis in the asymptomatic phase consists of correction of any secondary causes of hyperuricemia, including eliminating drugs like diuretics, low dose aspirin, and laxative abuse, limiting consumption of alcoholic beverages, gradual weight reduction for obese patients, and dietary restriction of purine rich foods. Foods rich in purines include organ meats like brain, heart, or kidney. These measures constitute sufficient therapy for many patients. Gout patients are often overweight and their blood pressure elevated. Some diuretic drug therapies for elevated blood pressure worsen and increase uric acid concentrations. They are best avoided. There are other antihypertensives available that are not diuretics that will not aggravate uric acid concentrations.

The prevention of gouty attacks depends on normalization of the blood uric acid concentration. The frequency and severity of attacks can be reduced by the prophylactic administration of small doses of colchicine once or twice daily. Chronic colchicine treatment does not reverse hyperuricemia and does nothing to prevent asymptomatic and progressive tophaceous disease. There is no doubt that patients with sustained significant hyperuricemia and who experience frequent gouty attacks of more than four a year will likely require long-term treatment with allopurinol or other drug. Although there are some foods that are high in the concentration of purines that are metabolized in the body to uric acid, they are uncommon in most diets and do not significantly affect the chance of developing gout. People rarely eat foods rich in purines like brain, sardines, anchovies, liver, sweetbreads, or other organ meats on a regular basis.

"Old wives' tales" always occur during the discussion of diet and gout.

Gout is often called the disease of the wealthy because of the potential contribution of rich foods to the cause. It is better called the "disease of plenty." During medieval times, individuals ate feasts and often developed gout. This has resulted in the belief that rich foods contribute to the cause of gout. Today, few Americans eat like that. The lead content of some homemade wine can result in kidney failure and elevated uric acid levels in the blood. This is a rare cause of gout and elevated uric acid concentrations.

When getting ready for a trip away from home, gout patients should pack their medicine before anything else. An attack of acute gout away from home is a difficult situation, but the rapid and early institution of either colchicine or an anti-inflammatory can stop it quickly. On occasion, attacks are resistant to traditional antigout medications, so that either intra-articular or oral steroids are utilized for a short while. Oral steroids like methylprednisolone (Medrol Dosepack) are used for a few days, or even prednisone for extended periods of time. Usually oral steroids can be avoided or eventually discontinued.

Acute attacks of gout, regardless of the area involved, including the joint, bursa, or tendon are extremely painful. The pain of acute attacks compares to having surgery without anesthesia.

The treatment of most gout is quick and gratifying. There are few excuses for chronic tophaceous gout in modern times. Individuals allergic to the medicine or who do not comply have difficulty lowering their uric acid concentrations.

Pseudogout

Pseudogout is an acute self-limiting arthritis similar to the acute inflammation occurring with gout. It is predominately a disease of the elderly, and targets the knees, wrists, shoulders, and hips. Acute episodes are caused by the body's reaction to crystal deposits within the joint and cartilage. The difference between pseudogout and gout is the type of crystals and the specific joints affected. The chronic form of this arthritis has a strong association with osteoarthritis. The clinical syndrome is associated with intra-articular calcification deposition seen on x-ray called chondrocalcinosis. It is referred to as calcium pyrophosphate disease (CPPD).

There is a female preponderance of patients and a striking association with aging. Chondrocalcinosis is most unusual under the age of fifty. Numerous metabolic diseases occur concurrently, including diabetes, Paget's disease, thyroid disease, hemachromatosis, and hyperparathyroidism.

Pseudogout is the most common cause of acute monoarthritis or arthritis of one joint in the elderly. Acute arthritis or acute pseudogout may be the only symptom of asymptomatic calcification of cartilage seen on x-ray. The cartilage of the joint becomes saturated with calcium crystals. It is unclear why the calcium deposition leaves the cartilage in some individuals and enters the joint space to precipitate inflammation in others. The knee by far is the most common joint involved. A typical attack occurs rapidly and without warning. The attack is characterized by severe pain and inflammation. The joint is swollen, red, warm, and painful. Attacks usually resolve over several days. Most attacks occur spontaneously.

In chronic forms of the arthritis, symptoms are often restricted to a few joints, though single or polyarticular forms occur too. Attacks may be superimposed on chronic pain, stiffness, and limitation of movement. Inflammatory features are easily confused with rheumatoid arthritis. Severe destructive arthritis occurs on occasion. Osteoarthritis is a common accompaniment. Involvement of the knee often results in fixed flexion deformities of the joint that makes ambulation difficult. For this reason, during acute attacks pillows under the knees should be avoided, even though this is a comfortable position.

In the elderly population pseudogout is to the knee like the gout is to the big toe.

Removal of the fluid from a swollen joint provides an opportunity to demonstrate pseudogout crystals. The crystal is characteristically different than the crystal of gout and even with a polarizing microscope it is difficult to see. Rheumatologists are trained to recognize and identify the crystal.

Calcification of cartilage is seen faintly on standard x-rays, especially in the fibrocartilage of the knee or wrists, but also in hyaline cartilage of the knee, shoulder, or hip.

Treatment

The goal of medical management is to reduce symptoms quickly, identify and verify the cause as pseudogout, and to mobilize the patient as early as possible. Simple oral analgesics and most NSAIDs give relief. Colchicine is rarely used. Intra-articular or oral steroids are necessary on occasion. Unlike gout, there is no specific therapy. Treatment of any underlying metabolic disease does not necessarily influence outcome. Changes or avoidance of foods in the diet have no effect on pseudogout.

Seronegative Spondyloarthropathy

Spondyloarthropathies share a number of similar features. Ankylosing spondylitis, psoriatic arthritis, Reiter's syndrome, and the arthritis associated with inflammatory bowel disease like Crohn's disease and ulcerative colitis are more common in men and have a tendency to involve the spine. They are systemic illnesses because they affect other organs than the joints such as the eyes, mouth, skin, kidneys, heart, and lungs. The blood test for rheumatoid arthritis is characteristically negative; therefore, these diseases are referred to as seronegative. Since the spine is involved with an inflammatory process, these types of arthritis are referred to as seronegative spondyloarthropathies. There is no definite laboratory test for diagnosing these conditions. The genetic marker or HLA-B27 occurs in over ninety percent of these people. There is a tendency for inflammation at the attachments of the tendons to bones called enthesopathy. These areas often calcify and are visible on x-ray. This calcification can complicate joint replacement.

"I know that I am not alone with this disease. The best thing I can tell anyone is I try to keep my chin up and deal with it. Try not to think of the pain. I just keep pushing myself. When I am having a bad day and I cannot do the little things in life that 35 years ago would have been so easy, I tell people keep a good attitude, laugh as much as you can and make others laugh, that helps cut the stress."

Charles Muhaw
Reno, Nevada

Ankylosing Spondylitis

Ankylosing spondylitis (AS) is a form of arthritis primarily affecting young men. Women develop the disease less often. Spinal involvement is usually the first manifestation. Inflammation of the spine develops slowly in young people during their late teens and early twenties, usually ascending the spine over many years. The first symptom may be a low backache. Many people mistakenly attribute these symptoms to excessive bending, lifting, sitting, or sleeping awkwardly. Unlike most low back pain, the pain associated with AS is worse during periods of rest or inactivity. These patients actually do better with exercise. Characteristic bone forma-

tions, syndesmophytes join adjacent vertebras. These bone formations are different than those seen in osteoarthritis. The inflammation stiffens the spine and results in loss of flexibility. Syndesmophytes can be so extensive that the spine takes on a bamboo appearance on x-ray. Inflammation and then fusion of the sacroiliac joints are the first area of involvement. The fusion of the sacroiliac joints can be seen on x-ray or by CT scanning. Over a long period of time posture becomes stooped. For some this can be severe. Stooped posture can be corrected, but only after difficult and extensive spinal surgery. A peripheral arthritis of the joints of the arms and legs may occur. Systemic symptoms include inflammation of the anterior portion of the eye called iritis, inflammation of the upper lung fields easily confused with tuberculosis, and interference with the electrical conduction of the heart detected on the electrocardiogram or EKG.

Psoriasis

Psoriasis is a noncontagious skin disorder that appears as an inflamed rash and skin lesions covered with silvery white scales. These patches occur in many areas of the body, but are more often in the scalp, elbows, knees and/or lower end of the low back. Rash can be confined to the scalp only and sometimes must be looked for carefully within the hairline. Patients are not always aware of the psoriasis in the scalp and contribute the rash to dandruff. Psoriasis commonly affects the nails and causes pitting or lifting of the nails called onycholysis. The rash has different variations and does not follow a predictable course. The swelling of the fingers and/or toes because of the arthritis gives an appearance of sausage digits. Swelling is not only confined to the area of the small finger joint, but the whole digit. No one knows what causes psoriasis, however, there may be a genetic defect of the immune system. About six million Americans are affected by psoriasis, women and men equally. The arthritis occurs in a small percentage of those people with rash, about twenty to thirty percent, but can occur before the rash is obvious. Activity of the arthritis correlates well to the activity of the skin rash. Gout, which is not a seronegative spondyloarthropathy, is more common in those individuals with psoriasis. The laboratory tests and markers for other forms of rheumatic illness are negative. Psoriatic arthritis has several forms.

Controlling the skin rash is essential to the treatment. Good skin care is important. Phototherapy may be helpful. Many of the patients do better in the summer. Systemic steroids are typically avoided. The response to oral steroids is limited and sometimes leads to the need for larger and larger doses. Oral steroids complicate the disease. Topical steroids applied to the skin are useful for the skin rash, but not the arthritis. Methotrexate

has an important role and is beneficial both for the skin and for arthritis. Gold injections and oral antimalarials have been used to treat the arthritis. On occasion, both can aggravate the rash. Newer anti-TNF agents are being explored.

FORMS OF PSORIATIC ARTHRITIS

- A symmetrical polyarthritis like rheumatoid arthritis

- An oligoarthritis that is asymmetrical; less than five joints

- Involvement limited to the last joints of the fingers, occurs more often when the fingernail is involved with psoriasis; this is the most common form

- A seronegative spondyloarthropathy, involvement of the spine; about five percent of the psoriasis patients

- Arthritis mutilans, a severely destructive form of arthritis; significant changes evidenced by x-ray

---

Reiter's Syndrome

Reiter's syndrome includes inflammation of the joints, eyes, and the genital, urinary, or gastrointestinal systems, and can occur following genital and venereal infection or bowel infection like dysentery. This reactive arthritis may be the immune system's response to the presence of bacterial infections in the genital, urinary, or gastrointestinal systems. Typically, the arthritis develops a few weeks after the onset of the infection and involves the knees, ankles, feet, or wrists. The infection may be chlamydia, salmonella, yersinia, or shigella bacteria. The source of infection may never be found; antibiotics are not always necessary. The arthritis is usually asymmetrical. Fluid accumulation in the knee can be extensive in comparison to other forms of arthritis. Inflammation of an entire finger or toe gives the appearance of a sausage digit, similar to other seronegative spondyloarthropathies. Inflammation at the insertion of the tendons results in tendinitis. Achilles tendinitis is common and causes swelling and heel pain. Inflammation of the eyes is usually confined to the white portion and is called conjunctivitis. The conjunctivitis is not painful. Other eye inflammation can be serious when it involves the iris. This is called iritis and is painful. Iritis can interfere with vision. Any portion of the urinary tract may be involved and may be entirely asymptomatic. Urinary tract involvement is discovered as an abnormal urine analysis, painful urgency or an uncomfortable feeling with urination, or even penile discharge. Sores of the mouth occur and go unnoticed, since they are painless. Inflammation of the large bowel precipitates diarrhea. Skin inflammation occurs on the penis or bottom of the feet. Fortunately, less common other areas of involvement can be serious, including inflammation of the aortic valve of the heart or the electrical conduc-

tion pathway of the heart. Treatment is determined by the areas of involvement.

Most of the arthritis and many other aspects of Reiter's syndrome will resolve spontaneously.

A number of patients will not require intervention. NSAIDs are helpful with the arthritis, topical steroid drops will help the eye most of the time, as do steroid creams with the rashes. The ophthalmologist should see those individuals with iritis, since this can result in blindness. Treatment with antibiotics is not always necessary. Those individuals with chronic evidence of inflammation, especially arthritis, find remittive drugs like methotrexate or sulfasalazine helpful. These drugs require close monitoring. Remittive drugs are often used when the arthritis resembles RA. Steroids by mouth or by injection can be beneficial.

Arthritis-Associated Inflammatory Bowel Disease

Inflammatory bowel disease (IBD) is a group of chronic disorders that result in ulceration of the small and large intestines. Most IBD is classified as ulcerative colitis or Crohn's disease. The inflammation of Crohn's may extend into the deeper layers of the intestinal wall, while ulcerative colitis is more superficial. Like inflammatory arthritis, IBD may be characterized by remissions and exacerbations. The most common symptoms include abdominal pain, diarrhea, rectal bleeding, weight loss, and fever. Arthritis occurs in a small percentage of patients. The arthritis occasionally precedes the bowel involvement. More often the arthritis relates to the activity of the bowel disease. The arthritis is usually in the lower extremity and may be migratory. Migratory arthritis moves from one joint to another in a short while, leaving the first joint without symptoms. IBD creates tremendous inflammation of the joint and is characterized by a severe swelling of the joint space. The arthritis usually lasts only a short time and does not cause permanent damage. Once the bowel symptoms are under control, the outlook for the joints is excellent.

Treatment

The therapy and natural course of each seronegative spondyloarthropathy has many things in common. People do better with exercise. Regular activity is important. Since the spine is involved, good posture is crucial. Periods of rest and relaxation are important between activities. Maintaining erect posture will help avoid stooping later. Sleeping on the stomach is preferred to sleeping on the back, but is difficult. Once a stooped posture begins, it becomes more difficult to correct. Pillows behind the knees should be avoided. While sleeping or resting, the knees should be kept as straight as possible to avoid permanent contractures. Swimming may be one of the best activities, since it encourages flexibility, deep breathing, and is an aerobic exercise. Anti-inflammatories are frequently used and, on occasion, second line antirheumatic agents in those individuals with a peripheral arthritis similar to RA. For those people undergoing major joint replacement, indomethacin is given to discourage extra bone formation or calcification around the new joint.

Scleroderma

Scleroderma is an autoimmune or collagen vascular disease characterized by the overproduction of collagen. This illness is known by other terms including "progressive systemic sclerosis" (PSS). Other forms include localized scleroderma or morphia and results in a hard patch of involved skin that may improve with time. Eosinophilic fasciitis is a variant of PSS. Scleroderma has important characteristics, although not entirely unique to PSS, including a characteristic color change of the fingers and hands (Raynaud's phenomenon), calcifications just under the skin (calcinosis), problems that make swallowing difficult, dilated small blood vessels visible under the skin, especially the face (telangiectasia), and tightening of the skin, especially the fingers (sclerodactyly). Scleroderma literally means "hard skin."

"My hands suddenly swelled. I was perfectly healthy up to that point. Now, I can't function normally. Daily things like putting on my socks,

brushing my hair or teeth are difficult. I have had to learn new and different ways of doing common things. My skin is tight. My fingers are contracting. It started in my hands and feet at first, then worked its way to my thighs. This disease has affected every aspect of my life. It has made me rethink my life and determine what is most important. I have come to a new awareness about myself and my character. I have come to realize the importance of family. I have become less independent and learned to rely on others. I have gained a spiritual strength."

Cindy Steeler
Reno, Nevada

Description

Excess collagen is deposited in the skin and other organs. Damage occurs to internal organs from the accumulation of collagen. Organs then get stiff and function poorly. Because small blood vessels are also involved, scleroderma is a collagen vascular disease. Collagen is found in the tissues connecting muscles to bones, but also other connective tissues like skin, cartilage, and ligaments. Lung or kidney involvement indicates a poor prognosis and encourages aggressive management. The cause of scleroderma is unknown. It occurs most commonly in young and middle-age women between the ages of 25 and 35 years of age, although men also develop PSS. The course is variable and ranges from mild disease to life-threatening if vital organ involvement occurs. It is chronic and usually lasts a lifetime. Occasional spontaneous remissions or regressions occur. It is estimated that as many as 100,000 Americans have scleroderma; even so, it is still an uncommon disease.

Clinical Course

CREST syndrome includes calcinosis, Raynaud's, esophageal motility problems, sclerodactyly, and telengiectasia, and may be a milder form of scleroderma. The letters stand for the most common symptoms of the illness. Calcinosis results in white hard lumps of calcium deposition just under the skin on the fingers or other areas. The calcium may ooze through the skin and release a chalky white material. Raynaud's phenomenon is a sensitivity to cold and precipitates color changes of the fingers and hands. Both hands and fingers or just a few fingers of each hand turn white then blue. When the hands warm up, the circulation improves and the skin color returns as the blood vessels return to normal. Raynaud's may or may not be painful. The blood vessels actually go into spasm. Nicotine or smoking and cold temperature changes like cold weather, refrigerators at home or work, and air-conditioned buildings aggravate the condition. Smoking must be absolutely avoided.

Common sense must prevail to control Raynaud's.

Some medications used for heart disease or hypertension help open up blood vessels and decrease the severity of Raynaud's (calcium antagonists like nifedipine).

Other skin changes of scleroderma include a hardening and thickening of the skin, especially the hands and fingers, arms, or face. Skin creases disappear and the skin looks shiny and tight. When this occurs over the fingers, it is difficult to make a fist or bend the fingers. Severe scleroderma results in ulcerations of the fingertips. The fingers actually shorten. The skin becomes darkened. Telangiectasias result in small red spots on fingers, palms, face, and lips. They are not harmful or tender, but appear as dilated tiny blood vessels near the surface of the skin. If cosmetically displeasing, dermatologists successfully treat these with laser therapy.

Deposition of collagen in the lungs interferes with the normal exchange of oxygen. Shortness of breath and eventually heart failure occurs. Blood pressures on the right side of the heart increase as the heart pushes blood through a diseased and stiff lung (pulmonary hypertension). Whenever the heart or lungs are involved, functional disability is significant and lifestyle hampered. Increasing shortness of breath, persistent cough, or chest pain necessitate evaluation and, on oc-

casion, additional medicines or the need for supplemental oxygen.

Swollen joints are not as common as is a puffiness of the hands and feet. Arthritis and muscle weakness is part of this disease. Fatigue will often follow these symptoms. When the skin and other tissues around a joint become too tight, the joint becomes difficult to move remaining permanently bent or flexed, resulting in a contracture. Leathery rubs can be heard as the tendons move over the joints. Early PSS mimics RA.

Collagen vascular diseases may involve the salivary or lacrimal glands. This leads to a decrease of secretions in the eyes and mouth. It is difficult to make tears or saliva. Dry mouth results in increased dental cavities and eye irritation. Meticulous dental and eye care become even more important as preventive measures.

The entire gastrointestinal tract can be involved in scleroderma. If the lower esophagus muscles are involved, swallowing difficulties and/or acid reflux occurs. Reflux causes heartburn. The constant reflux of acid into the esophagus can result in a stricture of the esophagus or narrowing before entering the stomach. Besides heartburn, swallowing is difficult and can result in vomiting or weight loss. Elevating the head of the bed, not lying down immediately after meals, and eating small meals are helpful preventive measures to avoid reflux problems. Medicines to prevent acid formation or antacids are aids to minimize chronic inflammation that causes the irritation of the esophagus. Weakness of the muscles of the colon's wall results in bloating, diarrhea, or constipation, nausea and vomiting, and even weight loss. Large-mouthed outpouches of the colon called diverticula occur.

Collagen deposition in the vessels of the kidney creates or worsens high blood pressure (hypertension). This is an important prognostic indicator; it can result in significant complications, and shorten lifespan. Hypertension cannot be ignored and should be treated quickly and aggressively.

The diagnosis of scleroderma is confirmed during a physical examination. Antibody tests are helpful. Some of these tests like the Scl-70 are specific to the systemic form of the disease. Routine laboratory tests evaluate various organ functions. The biopsy of the skin is characteristic, but not often necessary. Other tests determine involvement of the lungs, heart, esophagus or intestines, but are not necessarily pathonomonic. Looking at the capillaries of the nailfolds is useful to some experts.

Treatment
Early studies suggested that scleroderma improves with minocycline, a common antibiotic. The mechanism by which this occurs is unknown and remains to be proven. Minocycline should not be universally recommended at this time until more definitive studies are completed. D-penicillamine theoretically breaks disulfide bonds between collagen and should help scleroderma patients. However, this too has not been scientifically proven to make a blanket recommendation that all scleroderma patients receive this treatment. Steroids are cautiously avoided in scleroderma, although are, on occasion, necessary. Finally, other immunosuppressive agents have been utilized, including methotrexate.

Osteoarthritis

Osteoarthritis (OA) is often called degenerative joint disease or DJD. It is also called "wear and tear arthritis." It is the most prevalent form of arthritis in the country, with more than sixteen million Americans having OA. About equal numbers of men and women have osteoarthritis. The onset and symptoms occur most commonly after the age of forty-five or fifty and are a major source of disability in the elderly, potentially equaling that associated with cardiovascular disease or stroke. Osteoarthritis disables two to six percent of the general population. Five percent of those over the age of fifty-five will experience osteoarthritis of the hip and half of these patients will ultimately require hip replacement.

"Osteoarthritis is the most common form of joint disease affecting women in the hands, and many older people in the large joints, particularly the knees and hips. As a physician, I have been frus-

trated with the treatment, since we have not been capable of reversing or repairing the damage to the cartilage. Fortunately, adequate use of pain medications, physical therapy, and joint replacement surgery help many patients to maintain joint function, good pain control, and productive lives."

Chris Scully, M.D.
Arthritis Consultants
Reno, Nevada

Description

Patients experience pain localized to the joint without the signs of inflammation seen in other joint diseases like rheumatoid arthritis. The pain is worse with activity and relieved by rest. As the disease progresses pain will occur with very little motion, even at rest. Pain in the hip is common at night. The pain is described as deep, aching, and poorly localized. Cartilage acts as a cushion or shock absorber that pads a joint between two moving bones; it is a very smooth surface providing movement of one bone over the other adjacent bone. Osteoarthritis occurs when the cartilage weakens or breaks down, leading to irregular rough bone surfaces and deformity. Defects of the cartilage are without symptoms. Pain comes on slowly as the joint space changes and pain fibers around the joint are irritated.

Most individuals over sixty-five have some evidence of osteoarthritis by x-ray.

Any joint may be involved, but the most frequently affected are the weight-bearing joints like the hips, knees, and spine. Involvement of the knee is likely to result in significant disability. X-rays are characteristic as compared to other inflammatory types of arthritis and show narrowing of the joint space, irregularity, but also bone growth or proliferation. Extra bone growth is called spurs or osteophytes. Blood studies in OA are normal including the erythrocyte sedimentation rate or ESR, a simple measurement of inflammation.

The incidence of OA increases progressively with age. Injuries, obesity, or overuse in sports or work activities put certain joints at higher risk for developing OA. Stiffness after sitting or periods of immobility characterize the first few steps of OA of the knee or hip. The stiffness usually lasts less than thirty minutes as compared to the stiffness of RA that may be prolonged or last all day. Joint stiffness may be exacerbated by weather changes. OA of the hip or knee is characterized by gelling of the fluid within the joint. The gelling of the joint fluid is responsible for the stiffness. No one knows why one person gets OA and another doesn't. Heredity may play an important role.

Hand

Heberden's nodes are the bony enlargement of the last joint of the fingers and are more common in women and likely to occur in female relatives. The last joint of the finger is called the distal interphalangeal joint or DIP joint. These firm or hard bony enlargements occur slowly over time, but may also come on more rapidly and be inflammatory. On occasion, they contain gelatinous material and form cysts. When inflamed they are painful. Later, they become large, but are usually not painful. The joint is stiff, but function is not impaired. Rarely do the DIP's require surgery. The middle joint of the finger is the proximal interphalangeal joint or PIP and OA in this joint is called a Bouchard's node. The base of the thumb, or carpal metacarpal (CMC), is a common area of OA involvement too. When it is tender, it is difficult to carry heavy objects, especially in the kitchen. OA of the thumb base results in a squared off appearance near the wrist. Transient relief after local steroid injections occurs. NSAIDs help and surgery on occasion is required.

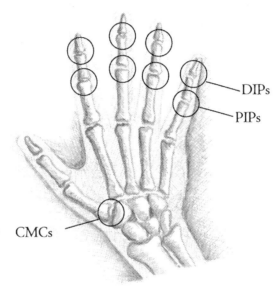

Figure Eight
Osteoarthritis involves several areas of the hands.

Hip

The pain of the hip is localized early to the groin or referred to the knee. This can be confusing. Limping is common. Crossing the legs may be difficult. Severe OA of the hip makes personal hygiene difficult. Getting off the commode can be impossible. In elderly individuals, hip replacement is needed to help with ambulation, but also to ease with transfers, self-care, and hygiene.

Knee

OA of the knee is aggravated by daily activities that require increased motion of the knee, especially squatting, climbing stairs, or walking. Walking down stairs is more difficult than going up. A grating noise called crepitation is often detected. If the knee is very swollen, fluid fills the front spaces of the knee above and below the knee cap or patella. Eventually, the fluid fills the space and goes elsewhere. Increased pressure sends the fluid to the back of the knee. This forms a popliteal cyst also called a Baker's cyst. The joint gets tight and results in difficulty extending the knee. The fluid no longer goes back to the front of the knee because of a "ball and valve" mechanism. This creates a one-way valve effect. The cyst gets bigger and tighter and ruptures. Fluid abruptly travels down the leg mimicking deep-vein phlebitis or a blood clot of the leg. It is painful and creates swelling of the calf and leg. Ruptured popliteal cysts are more common in inflammatory forms of ar-

above the knee. The muscles are then weak and the knee is at an increased risk for buckling or injury. Atrophy occurs in just a few days. Exercise takes months to gain back the muscle that was lost in such a short time.

A swollen knee or other joint is always more comfortable flexed, but propping of pillows or other supports behind a painful knee is

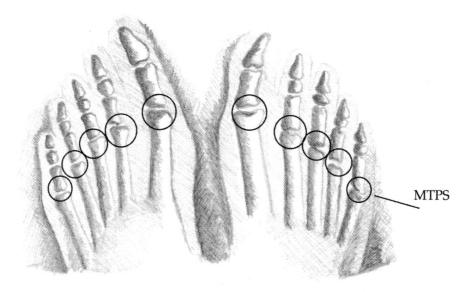

Figure Nine
The foot can be affected by both osteoarthritis or rheumatoid arthritis. The metatarsal phalangeals (MTPs) are often prominent on the bottom of the feet and make walking difficult. Prominent metatarsal heads are like walking on marbles.

thritis than osteoarthritis because more fluid is made within the joint spaces in those illnesses. Swelling of the knee or pain results in shrinkage or atrophy of the large muscles

discouraged. Keeping any joint in a flexed position for extended periods of time encourages a fixed deformity. A bent knee in a fixed position for extended periods may stay bent. This makes ambulation more difficult, requires more muscle strength, and puts tremendous energy demands on the person.

Variants of OA

Several variants of OA exist and include primary inflammatory forms of the small joints of the fingers that resemble RA. Diffuse idiopathic skeletal hyperostosis or DISH involves the spine with flowing calcification of the ligament in front of the spine. The calcification can be serious and large enough to interfere with swallowing when it occurs in the neck area. Most of the time, OA is relatively straightforward.

Osteoarthritis is associated with another form of arthritis called calcium pyrophosphate deposition disease, or CPPD. This form of arthritis is acute or chronic and typically involves knees, wrists, and shoulders. A crystal similar to the uric acid crystal of gout precipitates inflammation. It is referred to as pseudogout.

Treatment

There is no known cause or cure for OA. The treatment is both nonpharmacologic (without drugs) and pharmacologic (with drugs). Patient education is an integral part of the treatment program.

Treatment is tailored to an individual's needs to reduce pain, maintain and/or improve joint mobility, and limit functional disability.

Proper use of a cane on the opposite side of a diseased hip or knee teaches the patient to reduce the loading forces on the joint and is associated with decreased pain and improved function. The cane should be of a proper height or length. When the person is standing erect with arms to the sides, the top of a curved handled cane, or the level part if using a straight handled cane, should come to the level of the wrist crease.

Acetaminophen should be the first drug used in the treatment of OA. Later, NSAIDs and mild nonnarcotic analgesics form the basis of drug therapy. No drug therapy is known to change the course of disease or slow its progress. This is an area of research. Oral steroids are rarely used. Occasional intra-articular steroids provide rapid and significant relief. Steroid injections are justifiable for temporary and immediate relief, but should be done judiciously.

Since deterioration of the cartilage is central to OA, current research involves the biochemical factors of cartilage like collagen, protoglycans, and hyluronan. With very little scientific proof a number of unproven remedies have been suggested to improve the metabolism of cartilage. At this time, these remedies cannot be uniformly recommended. They include 5-adenosylmethione (SAM-E) and chondroiten and glucosamine sulphate.

Viscosupplementation, a series of intra-articular injections of hyluronan, helps return some of the cushioning effect of the joint fluid and relieves pain. Two preparations are available and include hylan G-F 20 (Synvisc) or hyluran (Hyalgan.)

The prognosis is good for OA. The disease progresses slowly and stabilizes without significant changes for years. Good lifestyle habits make a difference in the final outcome. Exercise helps maintain muscle strength, body weight, and general health. Swimming is best for those individuals with involvement of weight-bearing joints, but walking and even resistance exercise can help build muscle strength and improve range of motion. Common sense prevails when pain occurs with exercise. The expression "no pain, no gain" does not hold water, since pain is the body's best defense against further injury.

If you exercise the next day so much that you hurt more, you have done too much.

On occasion, joint surgery is necessary. Joint replacement of the major weight-bearing joints has enjoyed tremendous success. Arthroscopic surgery can now be performed in several areas and helps minimize recovery.

Inflammatory Muscle Disease

Muscle inflammation and weakness is called myopathy. Polymyositis is a disease characterized by muscle inflammation. There is pain or myalgias and weakness. The peak onset is between the ages of thirty and sixty, but it can affect children and people over sixty years old. Polymyositis (PM) usually affects the muscles of the shoulders, upper arms, thighs and hips. Involvement of the neck or chest muscles can make it difficult to breath, swallow, or lift the head. Systemic symptoms include fever, weight loss, general malaise, and less commonly joint pain. Muscle weakness can be profound or subtle. When the muscle inflammation is accompanied by skin inflammation the disease is known as dermatomyositis (DM).

"Diseases of muscle inflammation are frequently evaluated and treated by rheumatologists. This family of autoimmune diseases includes polymyositis and dermatomyositis. The main feature of these disorders is muscle weakness. The nature

of these diseases like most rheumatic disease is to be chronic and potentially disabling. Ironically, the medications utilized in the treatment may have side effects that initially worsen the weakness before it improves. It is crucial that patients suffering from these illnesses have access to and a long-term relationship with a physician knowledgeable and experienced in the management of inflammatory myopathies."

David J. Helfrich, M.D.
Rheumatologist
Pittsburgh, Pennsylvania

Polymyositis

Like other collagen vascular disease, patients with PM can demonstrate evidence in the blood of autoimmunity as measured by antinuclear antibodies or ANAs. These are markers for the disease. Prompt treatment includes anti-inflammatories, steroids, or immunosuppressants. Therapy can reverse or at least prevent progression of muscle weakness. Corticosteroid related problems occur frequently during treatment and contribute significantly to the functional disability reported by myositis patients. Large doses of steroids may actually contribute to weakness.

Dermatomyositis

Dermatomyositis is a similar condition to PM. It combines an inflammatory myopathy characterized by weakness and a characteristic skin rash. This disorder is closely related to polymyositis and may be part of a spectrum of the same disease. Both are considered connective tissue diseases or collagen vascular diseases. Each may be part of other connective tissue diseases like lupus. Dermatomyositis may be associated with malignancy, whereas the association with malignancy with polymyositis is perhaps coincidental. Both disorders occur in children.

At the time of diagnosis of dermatomyositis, there should be screening for cancer.

A *heliotrope rash* is a dark discoloration or a violaceous to dusky red rash with or without swelling in a symmetric distribution around the eyes. This may be obvious or subtle. Bumps over bony prominences especially the knuckles of the hand are elevated and violaceous and called Gottron's sign. The muscle weakness is primarily proximal and includes the part of the legs and arms closest to the body like the upper arms and legs. Initial complaints include weakness, fatigue, and an inability to do things that were taken for granted. Climbing stairs or getting off the toilet can be difficult or impossible. Inability to swallow suggests more serious involvement. Progression of disease may be slow or rapid over weeks and months.

Several laboratory abnormalities are typical of both polymyositis and dermatomyositis.

Muscle enzyme elevations in the blood like CPK, or aldolase are easy to measure, abnormal electrical conductivity in the muscles is measured by electromyography or EMG, and distinctive muscle biopsies characterize both diseases. The muscle enzyme elevation can be dramatic and is used to monitor the disease.

CRITERIA FOR THE DIAGNOSIS OF MUSCLE INFLAMMATION

- Proximal symmetrical muscle weakness
- Lab evidence of muscle inflammation
- Muscle enzyme elevation
- Abnormal electromyogram
- Abnormal muscle biopsy
- Abnormal magnetic resonance imaging
- Characteristic skin changes

Treatment

Several general measures are useful in treating patients with myositis. Bedrest is valuable. Rest must be combined with a range of motion exercise program to prevent contracture and preserve function for when the patient is stronger and better. The mainstay of treatment includes corticosteroids. Antimalarial drugs are useful in some patients. The overall prognosis varies, but intervention makes a difference and full recoveries are possible. Almost all patients will respond to high doses of steroids. As muscle enzymes improve so does the weakness. Eventually normal strength will return. Immunosuppressive agents like methotrexate are useful in those individuals with disease refractory to steroids or in those patients experiencing unacceptable side effects of steroids. Immunosuppressive agents allow lower doses of steroids.

Vasculitis

Vasculitis is an inflammation of the blood vessels, primarily arteries. The arteries can be small, medium, or large in size. Inflammation results in leakage of blood from the vessel, tender nodularity, and compromise and blockage of the normal circulation. If blood flow is entirely obstructed, tissue that the blood vessel supplies dies and gangrene results. In the connective tissue diseases, immune complexes of antibody and foreign antigen combine and deposit in the blood vessel wall. This complex causes inflammation and swelling which harms the vessel wall and interferes with the normal flow of blood. In small blood vessels this becomes important quickly and is painful. It can result in gangrene of the fingertips. Death of tissue results in the need for amputation or other surgeries.

"I don't feel ten years younger, I feel twenty years younger. From now on, I am going to do what you say. To tell you the truth, I now feel like living again." Comments from a patient during a discussion of her response to steroids for polymyalgia rheumatica to her doctor.

Margaret Savage
Reno, Nevada

Description

Vasculitis causes different symptoms depending upon which areas are involved. Systemic symptoms include fever, malaise, poor appetite, weight loss, and fatigue. Small red pinpoint or purple marks appear on the skin of the legs because the blood leaks from the vessel. These are described as petechiae. Larger areas of bleeding or bruising are called purpura. Infarcts are small painful black spots at the ends of the fingers or around the fingernails where skin has died. Pitting scars result on the skin of the fingertips. Other symptoms include joint pain, headache, behavioral disturbance, confusions, seizures, and stroke. Vasculitis of the nerves results in numbness, tingling, diminished sensation, or loss of strength. Heart attacks result as a consequence of coronary artery vasculitis. Lung involvement resembles pneumonia. Other areas of involvement include the eyes, kidneys, and intestines.

Forms of Vasculitis

There are different forms of vasculitis. A hypersensitivity vasculitis is associated with drug reactions or connective tissue disease. Several forms affect many organ systems and are life-threatening and are referred to as systemic necrotizing vasculitis. Other forms of vasculitis include Polyarteritis nodosa, Churg-Strauss syndrome, or Wegener's granulomatosis. These disorders involve major organ systems like the kidneys or lungs. Other forms of vasculitis differ depending on the organ systems involved or the size of artery inflamed.

Signs or symptoms of vasculitis are highly variable. The diagnosis is challenging. A biopsy of the involved tissue is diagnostic. Immune mechanisms in the bloodstream result in characteristic laboratory findings. Determining the exact extent of the disease is important.

Treatment

The treatment of vasculitis is the suppression of the inflammatory response or immunosuppression. Treatment includes steroids, cytotoxics, or immunosuppressive agents. Plasmapheresis is an alternative method to remove circulating immune complexes from the blood. During this procedure, blood is taken out of the body and spun in an apparatus that separates the different cellular components from the liquid portion of blood.

The liquid portion is discarded, since it contains the immune complexes that stimulate the immune response and inflammation. Cytotoxic drugs are given concurrently. These treatment regimes play an important role in the final outcome of the disease. Treatment is continued for prolonged periods of time to sustain a response.

Cyclophosphamide (Cytoxan) is the drug of choice for most forms of vasculitis. Daily dosing can result in bone marrow suppression and low blood counts. The dose is adjusted based on the results of frequent complete blood counts. Monitoring of the blood count is important. Suppression can be too great and the blood count too low. This puts the patient at risk for infection. Because all cytotoxic drugs can precipitate serious adverse effects, doses should be kept to a minimum to induce remission and obtain the desired effects. These drugs are associated with an increase incidence in some cancers. Bleeding of the bladder can be avoided by encouraging fluid intake, thus diluting the effects of the medicine in the bladder. Occasionally, large intravenous doses are given.

Azathioprine (Imuran) is another immunosuppressive agent. Although not always as potent in some forms of vasculitis as cyclophosphamide, it does have some advantages. Azathioprine is not associated with the gonadal suppression (sterility) that is seen with other cytotoxics, and doesn't have near the chance of inducing cancer. Blood counts can still be significantly suppressed and result in increased risk for infection.

Giant Cell Arteritis

Giant cell arteritis (GCA) is an inflammatory condition of large- and medium-sized arteries and usually affects branches of the carotid arteries. It is also called temporal arteritis. The carotid arteries are the major blood vessels that carry blood from the heart to the head. The temporal area is just to the side of the head behind the eyes.

GCA typically occurs in people over the age of fifty and is more common in women than men. This is the same population of individuals that develop polymyalgia rheumatica (PMR), and may be a spectrum of the same disease. Although they are likely to have the same cause, the reason why some people have only one syndrome and others both is still unknown. Frequently the two illnesses occur in the same individual. At least half the people with GCA also have polymyalgia rheumatica. Both conditions will often resolve spontaneously within about two years of onset and rarely return. In GCA symptoms include headache, especially over the temporal area of the head, jaw pain with chewing, fever, and scalp tenderness to touch or while brushing scalp hair.

Symptoms must be taken seriously. Some patients develop permanent blindness.

Treatment with oral steroids in high doses prevents visual disturbances, but must be started at the onset of the first symptoms. Side effects secondary to the steroids almost always occur. Occasionally, cytotoxic drug therapy and other immunosuppressives are necessary.

Polymyalgia Rheumatica

Polymyalgia rheumatica (PMR) is characterized by aching and morning stiffness in the upper portions of the muscles and joints of the arms and legs in a symmetrical fashion. It occurs in individuals over fifty years of age. The symptoms are often vague and difficult to describe. Fatigue and weight loss commonly occurs. Symptoms of PMR occur in two or three areas, including the shoulder girdle, pelvic girdle, and neck for one month or longer. There is almost always evidence of an elevated erythrocyte sedimentation rate (ESR). The onset may be abrupt, but in most instances the symptoms are present for weeks or months and eluded a definite diagnosis.

Comparing GCA and PMR

There is evidence of mild anemia in the laboratory or other mild abnormalities on the chemistry panel. The only significant laboratory abnormality is a markedly increased ESR, both in GCA and in PMR. The ESR correlates to the activity of the inflammation and response to treatment. The ESR relates to disease activity better than the patient's opinion or the physician's impression. It is followed frequently during the course of the disease. Extremely high ESRs are not uncommon and can be over 100 at the time of diagnosis (normal is less than twenty). The diagnosis of GCA is confirmed by a biopsy of the temporal artery. Characteristic changes are seen under the microscope. The temporal artery biopsy is a relatively safe and easy procedure done in an outpatient setting. Most often only one artery is biopsied. Biopsies are not repeated to monitor response to treatment, instead clinical symptoms and the ESR are followed. In GCA the abnormalities of the artery seen under the microscope are spotty and require a thorough examination of as long a segment of artery as available by the doctor. In PMR the arteries are not involved and need not be biopsied. X-rays show no specific findings.

In GCA treatment is initiated with high doses of systemic corticosteroids of at least prednisone 60 mg each day or greater and then tapered down slowly over months depending on symptoms and the ESR. Unfortunately, the treated population is elderly and the side effects secondary to steroids are significant, especially osteoporosis.

PMR is initially treated with lower doses of prednisone about 20 mg each day and then tapered in a similar fashion. A dramatic re-

CRITERIA FOR GIANT CELL OR TEMPORAL ARTERITIS

- Age at disease onset of symptoms greater than fifty years
- New headache and localized pain in the temple
- Temporal artery tenderness to palpitation
- Elevated sedimentation rate greater than fifty
- An abnormal artery biopsy

CRITERIA OF POLYMYALGIA RHEUMATICA

- Aching and morning stiffness
- Shoulder girdle involvement
- Pelvic girdle involvement
- Elevated sedimentation rate
- Mild anemia

sponse occurring overnight is characteristic. The next day a physician or nurse doesn't need to ask how the patient feels. Patients offer a spontaneous and immediate positive response. The results are so striking that patients resume their usual activities soon.

PMR often mimics RA, especially in those individuals with a negative rheumatoid factor. Both PMR and GCA run a self-limited course. Both will resolve. People treated for less than two years with prednisone have a high relapse rate. A small proportion of patients need steroids for an extended period of time. Most patients will experience side effects from prednisone. For the elderly population, osteoporosis is one of the side effects of most concern. A baseline bone density measurement should be done and calcium and vitamin D supplements started at the same time steroids are initiated. If steroids are continued for a prolonged period of time, bisphosphonates like risedronate (Actonel) or alendronate (Fosamax) should be started to avoid osteoporosis. Alternate day steroids are usually not as effective as daily oral doses. It is recognized that the complications of the steroids can be substantial in the elderly. Catastrophic complications of the disease are infrequent with treatment. Attempts should be made to taper the steroid dose slowly, while monitoring the ESR rate. During relapses in either disease, the ESR increases with the recurrence of symptoms. The ESR is the best means to monitor the disease. Both illnesses rarely occur when a normal sedimentation rate is measured in the blood.

Sjögren's Syndrome

Sjögren's syndrome is an autoimmune disorder associated with dry eyes and mouth and is called keratoconjunctivitis sicca. Primary Sjögren's syndrome occurs by itself and is not associated with other diseases. Secondary Sjögren's syndrome occurs with other rheumatic diseases. Most patients are women, although it can affect adults of any age or ethnic background. The Arthritis Foundation (AF) estimates that more than one million people in the United States are affected by this problem.

"My illness has never stopped me from doing anything, it has just been a big nuisance. My eyes feel gritty and eating dry crackers is almost impossible, but I have no joint pains."

Cindy Dressler
Truckee, California

Description

Although this can be a systemic illness like other rheumatic illnesses, Sjögren's syndrome is characterized more by the loss of tears in the eyes and saliva in the mouth than other rheumatic illnesses. Vaginal dryness also occurs. White blood cells (lymphocytes) actually invade the glands of the eyes and mouth and the production of fluids is lost. Fluid usually provides the necessary moisture for normal functioning. The glands are nonfunctional and eventually do not produce tears or secretions.

Saliva aids chewing and swallowing. When saliva is absent, both these activities become more difficult and cumbersome. The loss of saliva leads to tooth decay. Saliva contains protective mechanisms that fight bacteria and protect against tooth decay. Sometimes the patient experiences mouth infections. When saliva is absent, normal occurring yeast in the mouth or throat can thrive and cause thrush. Dryness in the oral cavities is a tremendous nuisance and results in cough, hoarseness, decreased sense of smell and taste, and even increased nosebleeds. In those women with vaginal dryness, intercourse is painful secondary to irritation.

The white blood cells infiltrate the salivary glands, cause pain and swelling and mimic lymphoma, a cancer of the lymph nodes. On occasion, a biopsy is necessary to differentiate Sjögren's syndrome from more serious diseases.

DRYNESS SYMPTOMS OF SJÖGREN'S SYNDROME
• Dry mouth
• Nasal dryness
• Vaginal dryness
• Dry skin

There are several ways to diagnose Sjögren's syndrome. Since treatment is often limited or conservative, invasive or more sophisticated testing is not always necessary. A lip biopsy is diagnostic, but uncomfortable and is seldom done. More sophisticated tests can be done to determine salivary gland function or tear production. Specialized blood markers detect antibodies that are more specific for Sjögren's syndrome, especially the autoantibody called Sjögren's syndrome antibody (SSA). Not everyone will have antibodies. Specialized eye exams look carefully for either the absence of tears or harm done as a consequence of dry eyes. Routine examinations determine systemic involvement, especially if the kidneys are involved or if there is other rheumatic disease like RA.

The cause of Sjögren's syndrome is not known. There is no cure or specific therapy.

Fortunately, this is not usually a life-threatening illness.

Treatment

The treatment of other rheumatic illnesses or associated problems is important and should occur first. Eye infections are treated promptly. Sipping water throughout the day is helpful for dry mouth. Sucking on sugar-free hard candies provides some relief and stimulates saliva production. Meticulous dental care is crucial and follow-up with dental professionals, including regular dental hygiene is important.

Treatment is designed to relieve discomfort and prevent any damage from the effects of dryness.

Artificial tears relieve the dry scratchy discomfort of the eyes during the day. Other products like lubricants or longer acting inserts are available. On occasion the ophthalmologist performs a simple operation that blocks the canal of the eye that drains tears. This helps retain tears and moisturizes the eyes longer. Vaginal lubricants help vaginal dryness and lessen discomfort. Pilocarpine hydrochloride (Salagen) tablets taken four times a day stimulate the salivary glands and production of saliva. The effect of one dose lasts only three to five hours. The most common side effect of this medicine is sweating. Other symptoms include chills, flushing, and frequent urination. Cevimeline (Evoxac) thirty-milligram capsules have similar benefits and side effects as pilocarpine.

Infections

Infections within a joint create inflammation characterized by pain, swelling, redness, and loss of motion within the joint. Several infectious agents can enter the joint. Infections within the joint are usually the result of infection elsewhere in the body, the result of the body's reaction to the infection *(reactive arthritis)* or the result of a suppressed immune system.

> *"Every year we travel to New England to visit with relatives. Last summer we took a side trip to tour Long Island. We played softball in a grassy field and found ticks on our clothing when we came home. Several days later I developed a rash and then arthritis. The doctors recognized my problem immediately, and sent me home on antibiotics. It all went away and has never returned again, thank goodness!"*

Raquel Snyderman
San Rafael, California

Description

Bacterial joint infections occur as a result of bacteria entering the joint from the bloodstream. Germs are carried to the joint via the blood. This occurs commonly in joints already damaged and weaker than healthy joints, but may also occur in normal joints and in young individuals. Bacteria enter through the upper respiratory tract like the nose, throat, or ears, through the gastrointestinal tract, or the skin. Surgical replacement of a joint puts the joint at increased risk for infection. Venereal disease, tuberculosis, streptococcal infections, and other skin infections can all result in infected joints at distant sites from the site of the original infection. It is not uncommon that a bacterial infection of a joint requires hospitalization and surgical drainage of the fluid from within the joint. Insertion of a needle and aspiration of infected joint fluid is diagnostic, but seldom therapeutic. Arthroscopy and synovectomy may be necessary. Acute bacterial infection of the joint is usually associated with high fevers and possibly shaking chills. The pain and swelling within the joint is severe. Individuals on steroids have a blunted or suppressed response to the infection, in addition to an increased risk for bacterial infection.

Other infectious agents or germs include viruses. Viral infectious arthritis includes forms of hepatitis, mumps, mononucleosis, or viral illnesses like measles. The rubella vaccine has been associated with a reaction similar to arthritis. Viral causes of arthritis are often a result of the immune system's reaction to the infection, rather than the virus actually being found within a joint. For this reason, as the virus infection resolves, most often so does the arthritis. Usually, there are muscle aches, headache, and low-grade fever. Antibiotics do not cure this form of arthritis.

Fungal infections are uncommon in healthy individuals, but more common in those with a suppressed immune status like intravenous drug abusers, cancer or cancer treatment, alcoholism, anemia, chronic illness, or acquired immune deficiency (AIDS). Infectious arthritis as a result of a fungus is the most resistant to treat and requires surgical intervention and months of medicine. Recurrence is possible. The infection is not always as inflammatory or obvious as the infections associated with bacteria.

Lyme Disease

Lyme disease is one of many bacterial infections that affect the joints. Lyme disease is a bacterial infection transmitted by the bite of an infected deer tick. The bite of the deer ticks carries the bacterium *Borelia burgdorferi*. The first reported cases occurred in Old Lyme, Connecticut. Now, most areas in the United States have reported Lyme disease, but it is more common in certain areas of the country, especially the Northeast and the Mid-Atlantic states, but also California and Oregon. It is important to be aware of the infection, its early symptoms, how it is transmitted, and protective measures to avoid tick bites. Most cases are reported in the spring and summer months when ticks are the most active and people are outdoors.

Early symptoms within a week of a tick bite include a flu-like illness in the spring or summer when the ticks are active. Achy joints or muscles occur with fever, chills, fatigue, and headache. At the site of the tick bite, a characteristic rash may or may not occur. It often looks like a "bull's eye"; a red ring with a clear center that expands and enlarges slowly over several days. Either the rash or actual tick bite can go unnoticed. Left untreated, Lyme disease causes more serious nerve or heart problems that mimic other conditions and make the diagnosis difficult. For most people, symptoms will resolve on their own within a few months without treatment.

Chronic arthritis resembling rheumatoid arthritis results as a consequence of Lyme disease. Only about ten percent of those infected will develop arthritis. In those individuals visiting or living in areas that are at higher risk, it is important to consider Lyme disease as a cause of arthritis otherwise unexplained, especially arthritis characterized by attacks in a few large joints like the knees.

Treatment with antibiotics is best started early and is generally successful. Treatment prevents more serious involvement. Laboratory tests are available to help confirm the infection in those individuals that have either physical findings or a history to suggest they are at risk for Lyme's disease.

PRECAUTIONS TO HELP AVOID LYME DISEASE

- Beware of early signs and symptoms, especially rash or tick bites.

- Beware of the small tick size; perform a tick check when coming in from outdoors, especially on small children, and shower when coming inside.

- Use tick repellent.

- Check small pets for ticks, avoid marshes or wooded areas when ticks are active, use tick collars or other repellents on pets.

- Wear protective clothing such as long-sleeved shirts or pants tucked into socks to avoid skin exposure. Light-colored clothing makes the tick more visible.

- Remove ticks quickly and carefully.

- Clear brush and grasses close to your home, especially in areas where children play.

The best treatment of Lyme's disease is avoidance of the tick bite, however that is not always possible with active outdoor living. Precautions and awareness of potential tick bites become even more important. The tick is very small and is easily missed, even so, small children and adults should inspect for tick bites after time spent outdoors. Using a tick repellent, protective clothing, and avoiding brush or other areas where ticks come in contact lessens the chance of an infection. Ticks are found in tall grasses in marshes and fields, or in the brush in wooded areas and are easily picked up on clothing or skin.

Parvovirus

Erythema infectiosum, or fifth disease, is the most common manifestation of parvovirus B19 infection in children. It presents as a mild febrile illness with a red rash of variable intensity. The early rosy to bright red "slapped cheek" appearance may be overlooked. Eventually a lacy, net-like redness develops that involves the face, arms and trunk. In adults the rash is less common, but infection involves the joints and resembles a more severe polyarthritis like rheumatoid arthritis. Evidence of previous parvovirus B19 infection in the blood is common among adults. Most forms of this arthritis will resolve without intervention and without any permanent impairment.

Rheumatic Fever

Rheumatic fever follows an infection with streptococcus bacteria, usually a sore throat. If the infection isn't treated early enough, rheumatic fever follows. Symptoms in children usually include fever, arthritis and inflammation of the heart. In some cases, this inflammation leads to heart problems. People who experience arthritis as the dominant symptom may experience recurrent arthritis flares later in life. As yet, there is no definitive laboratory test to identify rheumatic fever. The diagnosis is based primarily on the evaluation of clinical signs and symptoms. Although children are at most risk between the ages of seven and ten, adults also get rheumatic fever. In adults, arthritis is the most important manifestation, and in children the heart. Patients respond to high doses of aspirin for several weeks. Antibiotics are given to discourage a second episode.

Hepatitis

There are a number of viruses now responsible for hepatitis or inflammation of the liver. An associated antibody response by the immune system is responsible for a number of ill effects of the musculoskeletal system. Acute swollen joints often occur before there is clinically evidence of hepatitis. Hepatitis usually results in jaundice or a yellow coloration of the skin as the liver fails to clear bilirubin and other by-products of metabolism.

AIDS

Arthritis has been associated with the human immunodeficiency virus. Initial HIV infection may be associated with a flu-like illness. Some patients experience a painful articular syndrome. Whether Reiter's syndrome, psoriatic arthritis, or other reactive arthritis are more prevalent in HIV-infected individuals remains controversial.

Rubella

Like other viral infections, rubella is associated with arthralgias or arthritis. In most patients this is short lived, but in some it lasts for years. Joint symptoms occur just before or shortly after rash develops. Vaccines for rubella contain live attenuated virus. A high frequency of postvaccination joint pain, muscle pain, and arthritis is associated with the vaccination. Symptoms occur shortly after the vaccination, but then resolve spontaneously over several days. Occasionally symptoms last for prolonged periods of time.

Pneumococcal Disease

Pneumococcal disease is an infection that is caused by a bacterium. It is mentioned not because it is associated with arthritis symptoms, but because there is an added risk in people with arthritis and an impaired immune system. However, a vaccination protects from this potentially life-threatening infection. There are three general types of infection. Upper respiratory infections include the middle ear or sinuses. Lower respiratory tract infections include pneumonia. Other invasive infections secondary to the pneumococcal bacteria include sepsis or bacteria in the blood and meningitis or infection of the lining of the nervous system. Annually, pneumococcal infections account for more deaths than any other vaccine preventable bacterial disease and up to half of these deaths could have been prevented by use of the vaccine. All people with chronic forms of arthritis should have the vaccination.

Joints and Other Organ Systems

Joints connect the 206 bones of the human skeleton. Almost all bones are connected to the next bone by a joint. Each joint is classified according to the type of its movements or function. Most joints in the skeleton are freely movable, for example, the knee or finger. Joints of limited mobility include the area between the sacrum and pelvis. This allows movement at birth. Nonmovable joints do not move in relation to each other, like the joints of the skull. They are called sutures.

JOINT CLASSIFICATION BY TISSUE

- **Fibrous joints** are connected together by strong bundles of connective tissue. The sacroiliac joints are fibrous.
- **Cartilaginous joints** allow minimal movement. The joints between the vertebral bodies of the spine and the joints between the pubic bones are cartilaginous.
- **Synovial joints** are the most common in the human skeleton. They are freely movable with the bones separated by some space or joint cavity.

The cavity of a synovial joint is lined by a microscopic membrane or lining of cells called synovium. The cavity is filled with synovial fluid. The amount of fluid is small in the normal joint cavity, perhaps just a few drops and is clear or slightly yellow. Inflammation of the joint is synovitis, and is synonymous with the term *arthritis*. The synovium in rheumatoid arthritis thickens and goes from a few cell layers thick to hundreds of cell layers thick. Rather than a blockade, keeping fluid and cells from the blood out of the joint space, the synovium becomes leaky and allows fluid to come into the joint cavity. The joint appears swollen and painful. The fluid contains white cells, mediators of inflammation, and enzymes that promote chemical reactions harmful to the cartilage.

The typical synovial joint is surrounded by a fibrous capsule and forms the joint space. Each end of the bone is covered with hyaline cartilage, which forms a smooth glistening surface and functions as a cushion allowing the bones to slide against each other with minimal friction. Cartilage does not show up on a standard x-ray, but is more visible on sophisticated studies like magnetic resonance imaging (MRI). However, the size of the joint space is seen on x-ray and allows an estimation of the cartilage. Weight-bearing x-rays of the knee are useful to determine the amount of cartilage left in the joint space.

The movement of the joints depends on the muscles and tendons that are outside the joint space. The knee has fibrous bands or ligaments within the joint space that can be easily injured. Blood vessels are outside the joint space. During inflammatory arthritis or injury, fluid from the blood easily moves into the joint space and out.

JOINTS CATEGORIZED BY THEIR TYPE OF MOVEMENTS

- **Gliding joints** include the individual bones of the hands and feet.
- **Hinge joints** are molded to each other and move on a single axis as in the elbow.
- **Pivotal joints** allow turning of the palm of the hand face downward (pronation) and turning the palm of the hand face up (supination).
- **Condyloid joints** include the temporal mandibular joint. The TMJ joints close and open the mouth.
- **Saddle joints** include the base of the thumb.
- **Ball and socket joints** include both the shoulder and hip joints. The hip is weight-bearing.

Ankle

The ankle joint is weight-bearing and subject to the problems that this creates. The ankle is also subject to a number of injuries and/or fractures. Later in life, injuries can result in degenerative arthritis. The ankle joint is the site of arthritis in many inflammatory conditions like rheumatoid arthritis or psoriatic arthritis. Crystal-induced arthritis commonly occurs in the ankle joint. The ankle joint provides motion that is up and down and allows the stepping off and pushing off while walking or running. Restriction of this motion restricts these activities, especially going up or down surfaces or steps. The joint just below the ankle is the subtalar joint and allows *inversion* or *eversion*. These motions are movement inward or outward respectively, and when restricted or lost do not create much disability. It is awkward to walk with a fused ankle, but people with arthritis do very well with a fused subtalar joint and rarely miss the loss of motion. The subtalar joint is often harmed by rheumatoid arthritis and is painful.

High top tennis shoes, gauntlets, or braces provide important support. Unless the joint is completely fused, even a little motion during weight-bearing is painful. Ankle fusions are uncommon. Surgical fusion of the subtalar joint for rheumatoid arthritis is done frequently. Both operations require that bone from the pelvis be placed into the joint and the joint immobilized for several weeks while bone grows across the joint space. Once there is a solid fusion, there is no longer joint pain.

Elbow

The elbow is a unique hinged joint. Surrounding the elbow are several areas that may become inflamed, including the olecranon bursa or tendon attachments. Both tennis elbow and golfer's elbow are inflammation of the attachment of the tendons at the elbow. Tennis elbow occurs on the outside of the elbow and is most common, while golfer's elbow occurs at the tendon attachment on the inside of the elbow. Tendinitis occurs as a result of an injury, microtrauma, or overuse of the tendon. The pain is extreme, occurs at rest, and is aggravated with activity. Rest and local treatment of the inflammation are essential. A local steroid injection results in rapid improvement. Olecranon bursitis is acute inflammation of a small space at the elbow. This can swell abruptly and become very red, hot, and painful. Bumping the elbow can be enough trauma to cause acute swelling. On occasion the bursa becomes infected and requires surgical drainage. The bursa is inflamed in several other forms of arthritis like RA or gout. On occasion, the swelling is large and alarming in appearance. Rheumatoid nodules occur at the elbow in the area of the olecranon bursa and are hard moveable bumps. Tophi occur in the same area and can mimic rheumatoid nodules.

Because the hand is brought towards the body so many times a day, motion at the elbow is often preserved. Putting the arm out straight or at full extension of the elbow is not done often during a day's activities, thus this motion is not always preserved. Small and sometimes larger flexion contractures prevent full extension of the elbow. Fortunately, flexion contractures rarely interfere with function. Contractures make it difficult to reach the highest shelf in the kitchen, but most other activities are done without too much difficulty, especially those activities close to the body.

Occasionally, surgery is required, however, advances in elbow surgery have lagged behind hip and knee surgery. A person with severe arthritis of the elbow often functions with significant disability before resorting to surgical intervention. Elbow surgery is difficult because the anatomy is complicated. The demands on joint replacements are significant. The bones of the joint are small, the nerves and arteries are in close proximity, and there is a great deal of stress and leverage applied at the elbow. Most orthopedic surgeons prefer to wait as long as possible before doing a total elbow replacement in someone relatively young. A young patient will almost certainly outlive the artificial joint and require revision during his or her lifetime. An older individual with RA puts less demand on an elbow joint replacement. Risks and complications of total elbow replacement include stiffening following surgery, loosening of the prosthesis, infection, and damage to the nerves in close proximity. Infected olecranon bursae are usually surgically drained, rheumatoid nodules are not usually removed because they reoccur, and tophi can get smaller with medication rather than surgical removal.

Feet

The areas of the foot are divided into the hindfoot, midfoot, and forefoot. The hindfoot includes the heel, the attachment of the Achilles tendon, and plantar fascia on the bottom of the heel. Degenerative changes often occur in the midfoot. Unfortunately, the midfoot is a difficult area to treat. Perhaps, the most is done with the forefoot. The first joint of the big toe is subject to degenerative changes. The joint is weight-bearing and DJD creates pain with activities. Acute gout commonly involves the large joint of the big toe. Inflammation of gout is impressive and accompanied by severe pain, redness, and warmth. The skin peels just like a sunburn, since the inflammation is so intense. In rheumatoid arthritis, the second through the fifth joints at the base of each toe are commonly involved. The toes go up and the head of the other bone goes down. The forefoot widens making it difficult to find shoes that fit. Calluses occur on the bottom of the feet over the head of the bones. Patients describe walking on marbles. Resection of the heads of the metatarsals will shorten the foot, but provides comfort. Metatarsal bars or pads relieve some of the excess pressure in the area and provide comfort without surgery. Change of shoes, orthotics, or padding should always be considered before surgical intervention. The podiatrist is often helpful with these recommendations.

Several different surgeries can be done to correct bunion deformities, a deviation of the big toe towards the middle of the body. Angulation of the toes can be severe and at times toes cross each other. Pressure on the skin leads to sores or infections, besides the unwanted appearance, discomfort, or difficulty finding shoeware. Most surgery is successful; however, there is still a significant failure rate. Bunion deformities can reoccur.

Podiatrists are often asked to see patients with a burning discomfort between the third and fourth toes. Injection of local steroid or removal of small nerve tumors called neuromas provides dramatic relief.

Heel

Exquisite pain upon taking the first morning step, which gradually improves as you walk around, is characteristic of plantar fasciitis. Plantar fasciitis is more common in athletes because of their activities, in persons over age thirty, and those individuals overweight. "First step pain" is very distinctive of this disorder, even after just sitting for a short while. Heel pain comes on slowly. The first few steps taken after resting or getting up tend to be painful. The pain diminishes after a brief period of walking or with rest again. Plantar fasciitis is diagnosed by the physician during a physical examination.

Heel pain is common and in some cases chronic. Most individuals plagued with this problem can be reassured that it is not usually part of a more serious problem. With time,

and with simple and conservative measures, the problem resolves without any long-term effects. The most common condition associated with heel pain is lifestyle, that is, people without an underlying medical problem who are too active on their feet or weigh too much.

Heel spurs are often seen on x-ray, but do not always correlate with symptoms. The presence of a spur on x-ray doesn't necessarily explain the cause of the pain. There are many people with spurs on x-ray who do not have heel pain. Tests can be done to investigate other causes of heel pain, including fracture, infection, nerve entrapment, or tendinitis. The seronegative spondyloarthropathies are associated with heel pain because of Achilles tendinitis. Extensive diagnostic testing should probably be delayed for a brief period of time to determine if spontaneous resolution of the pain will occur. In most instances it will resolve on its own or with conservative measures.

There is no universally accepted treatment regime for heel pain.

Local modalities like heat, cold, or therapies by a registered physical therapist are appropriate. Weight loss is important. In some extreme cases, splinting or short leg casts help. Avoidance of strenuous activity is advisable. Patience and understanding are the key to conservative management. Stretching, a change in activities and shoe wear, and on occasion local steroid injections will provide some improvement in most people. NSAIDs provide further improvement. Other interventions are usually not necessary. Patients with refractory plantar fasciitis may require surgery, however, even this may not be entirely successful. Surgery should not be considered early in the course of pain.

Hip

Most forms of arthritis can attack the ball and socket joint of the hip. The hips are most commonly affected by osteoarthritis. Other inflammatory arthritis and injuries occur at the hip. Disease occurs in one hip or both. Some problems with the hip are congenital and occur at birth, but are not recognized until later in life. The blood supply to the hip is unique and easily subject to injury or interruption. Whatever the reason, if the blood supply is interrupted, death of the femoral head or the ball portion occurs and the joint is disrupted. This results in pain and limping. Early pain occurs in the groin, while later the entire area hurts. Pain may radiate down the leg and mimic knee pain. Fortunately, hip surgery is very successful.

Total hip replacement (THR), or arthroplasty, is an orthopedic procedure that involves the removal of the head (ball) and part of the neck of the femur along with the removal of cartilage of the socket on the pelvis. An artificial canal is created inside the femur and a metal prosthesis composed of a stem and small round ball for a head is inserted into the canal. The socket portion or acetabulum is enlarged and replaced with an artificial surface. These components are fixed firmly in place inside the bone, either with cement or by bony ingrowth into a porous coating on the prosthesis. This results in biological fixation. Bone will actually grow into the many porous areas of the prosthesis and secure it tightly into the bone.

THR is currently one of the most widely performed procedures in general orthopedic practice today. Since its introduction in 1969, it has proved remarkably successful in eliminating pain and restoring function of the hips. In some cases revision at a later date is necessary. Revision is more difficult than the primary replacement. There is less bone and the removal of the cement is difficult. The number of hip revisions in the United States is increasing steadily, since many of the early hip replacements are beginning to fail. Newer hip replacements will likely last much longer and for many individuals a lifetime.

More than seventy percent of THR's are done for osteoarthritis. These people have failed conservative management for pain and experience limitation in their activities of daily living. It is generally preferred that THR be done in those individuals over sixty. At this age the physical demands on the prosthesis are less. The longevity of the metal prosthesis approaches the life expectancy of the patient and avoids the need for revision. Regardless, this procedure is done at any age.

More than ninety percent of patients selected for THR achieve complete pain relief and improvement in function.

Even so, THR occasionally may be associated with complications. Patients are instructed to have realistic expectations of the degree of activity that is safely allowed. If abused, the prosthesis is exposed to wear, loosening, and a shortened life span.

In cemented hip replacements the cement is used to fix the femoral component in bone. In uncemented arthroplasties the prosthesis interfaces with the bone directly. In current practice the socket or acetabular component is rarely cemented. Uncemented components are fixed to the bone by bony ingrowth into a porous shell that surrounds the prosthesis. The most common metals that have been used are the alloy of stainless steel, titanium, and cobalt

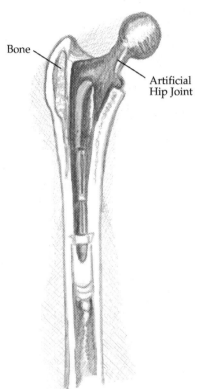

Bone

Artificial Hip Joint

Figure Ten
A total hip replacement actually replaces the end or ball of the femur.

chrome. They are biologically inert; no reaction occurs from the body. Ceramic materials have been used for the femoral head component, but there is some concern about the possibility of a brittle failure later. The cement is a self-curing polymer without adhesive properties and is used as a grouting agent to securely fix the components to bone. Cement implantation is done under pressure to ensure adequate filling of all empty spaces adjacent to the surface of the prosthesis. Noncemented total hip replacement was developed in response to evidence that loosening occurred commonly at the bone cement interface. Prosthetic devices that allow biologic ingrowth, that is fixation by bone ingrowth into a porous surface avoids the need for cement and has lower revision rates, making them more attractive in younger and athletic individuals. Postoperative courses are longer with uncemented hips, since full weight-bearing is avoided for several weeks. The surgical technique is more exacting. Despite all these efforts, loosening still occurs in some patients. Individuals with cemented hips are up and walking the first day after surgery.

Early complications of THR include possible fracture of the femur, nerve injury that usually resolves, dislocation if the patient is not compliant with instructions, and deep vein thrombosis which may or may not be associated with pulmonary emboli or blood clots to the lungs. Late complications include infection that requires removal of the prosthesis, extra bone formation around the site of the hip prosthesis especially in those patients with ankylosing spondylitis, and loosening. On occasion there is a leg length discrepancy. Shoeware compensates for leg length differences.

Simple precautions help prevent the chance of dislocation and include not crossing the legs, sleeping with pillows between the legs when in bed, not bending forward more than ninety degrees, and using an elevated toilet seat the first few weeks after surgery.

The high costs of this procedure are significant. Some are concerned that THR will not be allowed in all individuals in the future. The costs will come down as managed care limits length of hospital stays.

Knee

The knee has the distinction of being the most problematic joint. There are many reasons why our knees give us so much trouble.

INDICATIONS FOR TOTAL HIP REPLACEMENT

- Pain of the hip restricts activities
- Pain not relieved by simple arthritis medicine
- Stiffness or limitation of hip motion, including limping
- Pain in the groin at night
- X-rays confirm significant changes

The knee is the largest weight-bearing joint in our body. The knee is also the most complex joint. There are a number of internal structures within the knee that allow it to have so many motions. Extension and flexion allow us to run, walk, jump, kneel, bend, lean and generally abuse our knees. During the day our knees allow us to take thousands of steps and travel extensively throughout our environment.

Knee pain occurs as a result of constant abuse. Arthritis plays only a small part, although arthritis may be the result of injury and abuse over years.

Excessive weight adds to the abuse of the knees. It creates more problems than any other factor. Weight is supported by both knees. Exercise plays both a positive and negative role in the abuse and deterioration of the knees. Exercising the muscles in front of the thigh protects an arthritic knee, primarily by diminishing stress and pain of the knee. A swollen knee loses strength in the quadriceps muscles within a few days and gets visibly smaller compared to the other side just as fast. Jogging is a great aerobic exercise, but pounding forces while running on hard surfaces like sidewalks and streets is absorbed by the articular cartilage of the knee and are detrimental. Isometric exercises or tightening of the muscles in a straight leg fashion with or without weights while sitting strengthens the quadriceps muscles without aggravating the joint itself. It is not important to bend at the knee, but to raise the leg straight. Bike riding is fine if it doesn't cause pain or swelling and the seat is kept up to avoid extreme flexion at the knee.

The most comfortable position of any swollen joint is flexion. Flexion lessens the pain and discomfort, but encourages the knee to remain in that position. Frequent flexion is discouraged. A swollen joint should be kept straight most of the time, and then put through a full range of motion at least twice a day to preserve the greatest range of motion possible. It is difficult to walk about with a bent or flexed knee. This requires a very strong quadriceps mechanism. When the knee is weak, it is at an increased risk for buckling, further injury, pain, and discomfort.

Total knee replacements (TKAs) are done commonly and are almost as successful as total hip replacements. Osteoarthritis is the most common reason for knee replacement. Blood loss at the time of surgery is less than for hip replacements and blood transfusion occurs less often. Despite modern surgical techniques and early patient mobilization after surgery, blood clots remain a major complication of knee surgery. Deep vein clots in either the groin or calf are common following surgery. Fortunately, a fatal blood clot to the lungs is uncommon, but still remains an avoidable cause of death around the time of knee surgery. Preventing blood clots after knee surgery is difficult. If the blood is thinned before surgery there is a risk of bleeding at the time of surgery. There is a lack of consensus on the safest and most effective method to prevent blood clots. Current favorable methods include oral warfarin (Coumadin) therapy or injections of low-molecular weight heparins (Lovenox); neither require close laboratory monitoring as compared to other methods.

Low Back

Back pain affects almost one-third of the American population. Each American has an eighty percent chance of developing back pain during his or her lifetime. Under the age of forty-five, problems of the back and spine are the most frequent cause of limited activity and loss of work-time. It is estimated that over twenty-five billion dollars is spent annually in the United States on the treatment and compensation of low back injuries.

Back pain is known by several terms including sciatica, lumbago, pulled back, or the back going out. Much remains to be learned about each and every cause of back pain. For the most part, back pain is a result of non-specific muscle and ligamentous strain and will resolve with conservative treatment including rest, rather than spinal surgery.

In ankylosing spondylitis there is gradual fusion of the vertebral bodies of the spine over many years. This occurs in an ascending manner, starting in the low back then ascending to the neck. Rheumatoid arthritis rarely involves the low spine, but can affect the upper cervical spine.

The goals of therapy include relief of pain, gradual return to normal activity, and the prevention of recurrence. The single most important therapy for acute low back pain is bedrest. Recovery from back pain is frustrating and slow. Pain that spreads or shoots down the legs like a hot poker or electricity, pain that interferes with urination or elimination, causes numbness, is excruciating, or is associated with fever and chills requires consultation with a physician.

As pain eases, a program of exercises directed toward flexibility, strength, and tone of the back's supporting muscles must be started. Learning the movements and postures associated with aggravation or recurrence of complaints is important, in addition to learning proper lifting habits and low back mechanics.

The anatomy of the spine is complex. Each vertebral body rests upon the lower one. Each is separated by a disc that slowly dries out with age. As the disc deteriorates, it may move, compromising the space for the spinal cord or the nerves branching off from the spinal cord at various levels. Other portions of the vertebra overlap with the adjacent one to form facet joints. The spine remains flexible and allows multiple directions of motion. The spine is held together by several ligaments. As osteoarthritis develops with age, the bone develops spurs or osteophytes that compromise the space of the spinal cord or nerves as they exit. Nerves become pinched and cause severe burning, hot, or shooting pain down an extremity. In the low back this is often called sciatica, since it occurs near the sciatic area. Obesity aggravates low back pain secondary to facet arthritis.

Spinal stenosis results from degenerative changes of the central spinal canal of the back and the areas of the spine on the side where different nerve roots exit to supply the legs or arms. Degenerative changes result in narrowing because of bony or soft-tissue enlargement. This encroaches on the space for the spinal cord or the nerve as it exits the spinal canal. Spinal stenosis of the cervical or lumbar spine may require a surgical laminectomy to relieve the compression of the nerve structures.

Symptoms of lumbar spinal stenosis are vague and poorly localized. Leg pain on both sides is associated with numbness and weakness. The pain worsens with exercise and improves after short periods of rest. Symptoms are described as numbness, achy back or leg pain, a tingling or burning sensation, and buckling of the legs. Lumbar disc pain secondary to a herniated disc is differentiated by pain that decreases with standing or walking as compared to the pain that increases with spinal stenosis. Cervical spinal stenosis is associated with the radiation of pain down the arms like electric shocks and may be associated with headache or neck pain.

Medical therapies are utilized in those individuals with mild symptoms and no evidence of neurological deficit. Neurological deficits include loss of reflexes, weakness of the arms or legs, and loss of control of the bowels or bladder. If symptoms are more severe, incapacitating despite medical management, or neurological deficits are present, then further diagnostic studies are required to determine the level of stenosis. Medical management includes anti-inflammatories, immobilization, analgesics, rest, and the injection of steroids around the spine referred to as epidural steroids. With new technology, myelograms have been replaced by MRI or CT scans. Surgical intervention is necessary when there is no response to medical management.

Other causes of back pain include cancer, infection, fractures, or injuries.

Neck

Osteoarthritis affects the upper spine much like it does in the lower spine. Rheumatoid arthritis affects the neck in a unique way, especially between the first and second cervical vertebra. The second vertebra has a protrusion that extends up into and against the first vertebra. In severe RA this area becomes inflamed similar to other joints. The inflammation weakens the attachment of the two first vertebras and allows abnormal movement. When the head is flexed forward, the second vertebra can move compromising the space for the spinal cord. This abnormality can be severe and life-threatening. Fusion of the first two vertebras prevents this movement.

Shoulder

The shoulder is very different than other joints that are weight-bearing. The range of motion, strength, and function of both shoulders is unique to the shoulder joint. Unlike the ball and socket joint of the hip, the shoulder joint is more shallow and like a golf ball on a tee than a deep socket like the hip. Daily, the shoulder is subject to trauma and injury. Areas of inflammation include the bursa, tendons, or joint. A group of muscles surrounds the shoulder and make up the rotator cuff. These muscles maintain stability of the joint, but are subject to injury, degeneration, and tears. Tears are detected by ultrasound images, arthrography, or the injection of dye within the joint, and sophisticated magnetic resonance imaging. Tears of the rotator cuff are initially treated conservatively. Oral NSAIDs, physical therapy, and intra-articular steroids are all helpful. However, only surgery can repair a tear.

The tip of the scapula or acromion that forms the summit of the shoulder occasionally compresses the rotator cuff tendon and must be shaved down.

Any injury or pain of the shoulder can result in contraction and tightening of the muscles about the shoulder. Bursitis or any cause of pain at the shoulder quickly results in loss of shoulder motion secondary to tightening and contraction of the tissues and muscles surrounding the shoulder. This is called adhesive capsulitis. Within a few days individuals can't reach behind the back to fasten a bra, put on a coat easily, or place the hand in the back pocket of pants.

A total shoulder replacement (TSR) or arthroplasty is most often done due to arthritic change of the joint, in older individuals usually as a result of OA and younger individuals as a result of RA. Surgical advancements have greatly improved in recent years. A shoulder arthroplasty is effective in relieving pain and restoring functional mobility, but probably not to the degree and success of other joint replacements like the hip or knee. Fusion of the shoulder joint relieves pain at the cost of mobility and is most always avoided. If the rotator cuff mechanism is not intact, fusion may be the only option for relief of pain.

Sternum

The breastbone consists of more than one bone. Each of the connections between the bones and the attachments of the collarbone or clavicle to the sternum are joints and can be affected by arthritis. Swelling is visible and occasionally requires injection of steroids. Inflammation along the borders of the breast bone near the rib attachments results in chest pain called costochondritis. The pain of costochondritis can be severe and confused with the chest pain of a heart attack.

Wrist

Several important abnormalities occur at the wrist that are unique because of the anatomy.

Carpal tunnel syndrome (CTS) is common and occurs at any age. CTS is associated with other conditions than arthritis including pregnancy, hypothyroidism, or diabetes. It occurs more commonly in women than in men. Young patients are more often males. Work-related activities, especially vibratory or repetitive actions like carpentry, super-market checkers and scanners, meat, fish, and poultry processing are associated with CTS. Any inflammatory arthritis is commonly associated with CTS, but so is OA. Both hands may become involved. Symptoms come on slowly and are intermittent, although gradually occurring more often and eventually being persistent. Finally, difficulty with simple tasks like reaching for a milk carton or buttoning a shirt occurs. Late in this condition, the muscles at the base of thumb become small, soft, and weak.

CTS occurs as a result of pressure on the median nerve as the nerve and vessels pass through the carpal tunnel on the inside surface of the wrist. A ligament across the wrist covers the bones from the thumb side to the little finger and forms an arch or tunnel that allows passage of the nerves, artery, and veins to the fingers. Anything occupying the space results in pressure on the nerve. Pressure on the nerve causes pain, tingling,

and eventually nerve damage. The tingling sensation and numbness occurs in the thumb, index finger, middle finger, and at least part of the ring finger, and leads to weakness and a poor grip. Pressure on the nerve is just like hitting the "funny bone" at the elbow, which causes tingling down the forearm and hand. Without a healthy nerve, the muscles the median nerve supplies shrink, atrophy, and become weak. This results in loss of motor power, poor grip strength, and loss of sensation in the involved fingers. The symptoms are often worse at night, particularly while sleeping. Individuals wake up with their hand asleep, shaking or rubbing it, to bring the feeling back.

Area Supplied by Median Nerve

Figure Eleven

Carpal tunnel symptoms decrease sensation in the distribution of the median nerve as drawn here.

There are several ways to determine if symptoms are the result of CTS. Often, it is obvious to the physician and treatment can be undertaken without definitive diagnostic testing. Gentle tapping over the median nerve at the area of the carpal tunnel will duplicate the symptoms. Holding both hands against each other in flexion or extension for several seconds will also duplicate the symptoms. Measuring the nerve's ability to send an electrical impulse through the median nerve to the muscles can be determined by nerve conduction studies (NCV), and is useful if surgery is contemplated and the diagnosis must be assured. This test places small needles on both sides of the wrist and sends a small electrical shock across the wrist that can be measured. If there is a block, the electrical impulse on the other side will be diminished. It is well tolerated and really not painful. Nerve conduction tests are done by medical specialists. Blood tests examine for other medical conditions.

Treatment should be conservative and simple. Initially, changing work activities helps. Rest periods, alternating tasks, or modifying jobs may resolve the problem. Wearing a protective splint at work or night is helpful. This protects from excessive motion at the wrist and places the wrist in a comfortable resting position. Splints can be purchased at the drugstore. If inflammation is a major part of the cause, a local steroid injection into the carpal tunnel space near the nerve may be helpful and can solve the problem. Oral anti-inflammatories help reduce the swelling and increased pressure within the carpal tunnel space. Symptoms occurring during pregnancy usually resolve after the baby is delivered. Thyroid replacement will benefit people with low thyroid and symptoms of CTS.

The symptoms of CTS may continue for years. Persistent symptoms result in irreversible weakness of the hand. Early symptoms are occasional, but as time goes on the symptoms become more constant and more severe. After conservative therapy or modification of activities, surgery is necessary to avoid permanent damage to the nerve and the muscles it supplies. The surgical procedure is called a carpal tunnel release. The ligament trapping the median nerve is cut and the pressure on the nerve released. This is done as an outpatient procedure and in some individuals accomplished through a scope, rather than a long incision of the wrist. Recovery is complete and rapid, allowing the individual to return to usual activities after several weeks. Second surgeries for CTS are most unusual, although both wrists may have to be done. The treatment of carpal tunnel symptoms can be summarized into a list.

TREATMENT OF CARPAL TUNNEL SYNDROME

- Avoidance of repetitive activities or stress at the wrist
- Rest, splinting, the use of anti-inflammatories, local steroid injection
- Treatment of other medical conditions
- Surgical release of the ligament at the wrist

Hand

The changes of the hand in RA are characteristic and described under the chapter for rheumatoid disease. Different characteristic changes are noted in OA and are described in the chapter on degenerative arthritis. The tophi of gout can occur on the fingers and exude white chalky material of urate crystals. Tenosynovitis or tendinitis occurs just above the wrist on the side of the thumb and is described in the chapter on tendinitis. Fingers will trigger if the tendon thickens or gets a bump that catches. This is painful, but usually responds to a local steroid injection.

Eye

Autoimmune diseases deposit autoantibodies in different tissues. Depending on where that happens determines the disease. It is difficult to find an inflammatory arthritis that doesn't involve the eyes.

About one third of patients with rheumatoid arthritis have Sjögren's syndrome. Tear production is reduced and results in a gritty feeling of dryness, irritation, and burning. Most people relieve their symptoms with artificial tears to lubricate the eyes. Dry eyes are a terrible nuisance and result in infections on occasion. A more serious and less common problem is acute irritation and inflammation of the blood vessels in the white of the eye or sclera called scleritis. This occurs with more serious arthritis. The eye becomes red and painful. Topical steroids relieve the inflammation, pain, prevent corneal damage, and loss of vision. The sclera becomes thinned, and on rare occasions, requires surgery to prevent rupture.

The eye complications of giant cell arteritis appear early in the disease, but fortunately, affect only a small percentage of individuals. Steroids prevent loss of vision and blindness.

Inflammation of the iris or colored part of the eye is called iritis. If iritis is left untreated, it can lead to visual loss. The condition can resolve, recur, or become chronic.

Several medications cause problems with the eye. Antimalarials require close monitoring by an eye physician. Despite concerns about toxicity, antimalarials are among the safest of drugs used to treat rheumatoid arthritis and other rheumatic disease. Regular and frequent eye examinations detect early damage to the back of the eye. Antimalarials are discontinued before irreversible damage or impairment of vision occurs.

Corticosteroids put patients at risk for developing cataracts and glaucoma. Both conditions are already common in older patients. Cataracts result in a cloudiness of the eye's lens and blurred vision. People using steroids have accelerated cataract formation. A cloudy lens can be removed and replaced with a plastic lens. Replacement of a new lens and removal of the cataract restores near normal vision.

Glaucoma results in increased pressure and fluid within the eye. Increased pressure can hurt the eye and result in visual impairment. Medication in the form of eye drops reduces the production of fluid and the pressures.

Heart

The heart is involved in several ways with rheumatic disease. Inflammation of the heart sac or pericarditis mimics chest pain like a heart attack. Fluid accumulates in the space between the heart and the sac, and is called a pericardial effusion. If the fluid accumulates quickly or in large amounts, the heart is restricted and fails. Symptoms include shortness of breath or chest pain and eventually edema in the lower legs occurs. Anti-inflammatory medicine prevents accumulation of the fluid and allows the fluid to be reabsorbed. If unsuccessful, aspiration through a small needle or surgery can alleviate the pressure and restriction of the heart. Quick decisions and actions are required. Other causes of pericarditis and fluid accumulation include infection or even tumor.

Other areas of the heart can become inflamed and dysfunction. Interference of the electrical conduction system of the heart, abnormal growths or thickening of heart valves, and even inflammation of the coronary arteries all occur in rheumatic disease.

Lung

Involvement of the lung with rheumatic disease takes several forms, including inflammation of the lining of the chest wall or covering of the lungs called pleurisy, spots within the depth of the lungs called pulmonary nodules which mimic tumor or infection, or inflammation within the depth of the lung tissues called pulmonary infiltrates. Infiltrates appear like pneumonia. Inflammation of the lungs results in scarring or fibrosis of the lung field. Fibrosis interferes with oxygen exchange and results in shortness of breath and right heart failure. Oxygen is often necessary. The treatment and prognosis of pulmonary fibrosis is poor. Whenever the lungs are involved with autoimmune disease, there is always an increased susceptibility for infection and sometimes unusual infections.

Skin

All collagen vascular disease is associated with rashes or other skin ailments. Some primary skin problems are associated with arthritis. Inflammation of arteries within the skin is called cutaneous vasculitis. Compromising the blood supply results in skin death or gangrene and sloughing or ulceration of the skin. Severe involvement can result in amputation, other surgeries, and even death. Skin infections are more common in all rheumatic illnesses. Shingles or herpes zoster and fungal infections like monilia are not uncommon.

Other Rheumatic Illnesses

Other rheumatic illnesses must be briefly described. Numerous syndromes and unique problems related or associated with rheumatic illness have now been described.

Antiphospholipid Syndrome

The combination of increased blood clotting or thrombosis, miscarriages, and low platelet counts make up the antiphospholipid antibody syndrome. This syndrome was first described in lupus patients. Fifty percent of patients with these antibodies do not have lupus. Studies suggest that the presence of antiphospholipid antibodies increase the future risk of thrombotic events like deep venous thrombosis, stroke, gangrene, and heart attack. Blood tests easily detect the presence of antiphospholipid antibodies. There are several different antiphospholipid antibodies. Most commonly measured in the laboratory are the lupus anticoagulant and anticardiolipin antibody. These antibodies react with phospholipid, a fat molecule that is part of a normal cell membrane. Because of this phenomenon patients develop a false positive test for syphilis even though they have never had this infection.

Anticardiolipin antibodies have been found to be present in some pregnant women with lupus. These same women have more miscarriages. Excess blood clotting in the placenta is responsible for miscarriages and must be prevented if the pregnant lupus patient is to carry the fetus to full term.

Much remains to be learned about the treatment of this problem. There are a number of methods to thin or anticoagulate the blood and eliminate the risk for thrombosis or clotting. Even though a woman has antibodies, if there has never been any abnormal blood clotting, treatment is usually not necessary. However, once there has been a complication of the antiphospholipid syndrome, "thinning" of the blood by one method or another is indicated. This is accomplished not to dissolve the current clot, but to prevent future clotting. Aspirin in small amounts, warfarin (Coumadin), or injections of heparin, anticoagulate the blood. One baby aspirin interferes with the stickiness of platelets for weeks. Platelets circulate in the blood and plug up holes and sites of bleeding. Since they are so sticky, they clump together easily and plug bleeding sites. Both warfarin and

heparin block the clotting process, and in most cases provide much more complete and thorough thinning of the blood than aspirin. They also increase the risk of bleeding more than aspirin, and therefore, require close monitoring by a physician.

If a woman with lupus has antiphospholipid antibodies and is pregnant for the first time, or has had normal pregnancies in the past, no treatment is advised. If the same woman has a history of miscarriages, several different treatment regimes are recommended including aspirin, steroids, or injections of the blood thinner, heparin. All pregnancies in women with lupus who have antiphospholipid antibodies should be considered at high risk for miscarriage, premature delivery, or stillbirth.

Breast Implants and Connective Tissue Disease

The association of silicone breast implants (SBIs) with a variety of connective tissue diseases (CTDs) is widely reported and publicized. In spite of this, physicians, the public, and implant recipients do not have a clear understanding of whether SBIs are truly associated with the development of connective tissue disease. It remains a medical controversy.

Years ago, silicone was perceived as a safe, inert material, and ideal for the use of breast augmentation. It is now clear that this initial perception was incorrect. All breast implant recipients develop at least some local reaction to the implanted material. This is called encapsulation and can sometimes be broken up by manual palpation of the breast. The most commonly reported systemic rheumatic disease in implant recipients is scleroderma. In scleroderma, the disease severity varies from localized skin involvement to diffuse systemic disease and death. The majority of SBI patients do not have scleroderma, but nonspecific symptoms such as fatigue, myalgias and arthralgias.

Silicone implants have been used for over thirty years. There have been about one to two million surgeries. Allowing for a long latency period between the exposure, surely more cases of connective tissue disease should have been reported. Of all the patients reported, few have sufficient findings to satisfy the ACR criteria for specific diseases. It is suggested that these patients have an undifferentiated connective tissue disease. Many appear to have fibromyalgia.

Large monetary rewards are offered to those who can clearly establish that silicone implants are related to connective tissue disease. Many of these cases remain in the legal system. Medical and legal issues muddy the waters and create confusion among experts. Whether or not removal of the implant or explantation will resolve a patient's musculoskeletal symptoms is debatable. Women with saline implants do not seem to be at risk.

Insufficient attention is paid to the concerns of over one million women with SBI who are currently asymptomatic. This controversy is far from settled. Currently, the FDA has banned further silicone breast implantation except under special circumstances. Silicone used in other medical devices is not associated with this disease.

Raynaud's Phenomenon

About ten percent of the general population has Raynaud's phenomenon (RP). Only a small percentage of RP patients will develop a connective tissue disease. The diagnosis of RP is based on observation. RP is most prominent in scleroderma patients, but can occur in individuals without any other medical problems. Blood vessels go into spasm and slow blood flow. This causes characteristic color changes of the hand or fingers. The skin will feel cold. As the finger is deprived of blood it turns white, and as the blood pools, blue or cyanotic. After the blood vessel opens up again, the skin turns red and painful. This occurs over a few moments or longer. It involves one finger, all the fingers, or other organ parts. It is precipitated by emotions and cold, including a cool room, and is severely aggravated by smoking. It usually does not result in any tissue damage, unless associated with more serious blood vessel problems. RP is more a nuisance than anything else, although it can be quite alarming in appearance.

Several treatment remedies are used to alleviate symptoms or lessen frequency. Mild uncomplicated RP is usually easy to control. Abstinence from smoking is mandatory. Any offending drugs should be discontinued. Avoidance of cold and abrupt changes in temperature is necessary. Insulated gloves or hand warmers are helpful. Avoidance of outdoor winter activities or cool air-conditioned rooms help. The institution of a calcium antagonist helps to open blood vessels and blood flow to the fingers. Although unusual,

finger ulcers require significant interventions when blood flow is severely compromised. More aggressive treatments include injections into the sympathetic nervous system or surgery. A spectrum of similar vasospasm phenomena results in mottling of the skin called livido reticularis.

HELPFUL MEASURES THAT MAY ALLEVIATE RAYNAUD'S SYMPTOMS
• Avoidance of cold
• Avoidance of stress and extreme emotions
• Strict avoidance of smoking

Ulcers

Ulcers of the stomachs are more frequent in the patient with arthritis than the rest of the population. A bacterial infection, *Heliobacter pylori (H. pylori)* is responsible for most peptic ulcers of the gastrointestinal tract, regardless whether these individuals have arthritis or not. NSAIDs are responsible for twenty-five percent or more of the stomach ulcers not related to this infection.

Infection

H. pylori is a spiral-shaped bacterium that screws itself into the lining of the upper GI tract, usually the stomach or upper section of the small intestine or duodenum. Researchers are unclear how the bacteria is transmitted, but the diagnosis is relatively easy and the treatment effective.

There are several ways to test for *H. pylori* infection, including a serum or blood antibody test, a biopsy of the stomach wall at the time of an upper endoscopy, and a breath test. Other diagnostic tests are still preliminary and under investigation.

H. pylori-induced ulcers are generally confined to the upper small intestine just following the stomach, while NSAIDs cause their damage in the stomach itself. *H. pylori*-induced ulcers are usually symptomatic, while NSAID-induced ulcers may not cause symptoms at all.

NSAIDs

NSAIDs work by blocking or limiting the production of prostaglandins. Research has demonstrated that "good" and "bad" prostaglandins exist. The "bad" prostaglandins contribute and play an important role mediating the inflammation and pain of arthritis, but "good" prostaglandins, like those in the lining of the stomach wall are protective. "Good" prostaglandins do many of the normal housekeeping functions necessary to keep the body healthy. Prostaglandins in the stomach wall protect the lining of the stomach wall from acid secretion. The "bad" prostaglandins are often induced by infection or disease. The suppression of prostaglandins by NSAIDs is considered beneficial and is responsible for benefits to the arthritis patient, including pain relief. More must be learned about NSAIDs' and prostaglandins' role in the body.

Most current NSAIDs given to treat pain and inflammation of arthritis cannot differentiate "good" from "bad" prostaglandins. Therefore, even NSAIDs available over the counter inhibit the production of both. NSAIDs work by blocking the activity of the enzyme cycloxygenase (COX). This enzyme is necessary for the formation of prostaglandins. Without this enzyme, "bad" prostaglandins are not formed and less inflammation occurs; however, "good" prostaglandins are not formed either, and so the stomach is put at risk for injury and ulceration from its own acid. Researchers have discovered there are two different COX enzymes, COX-1 or COX-2. COX-1 is responsible for producing prostaglandins that are "good." These are the housekeeping prostaglandins that protect the stomach lining from acid. COX-2 is responsible for producing prostaglandins that are "bad" and cause the inflammation and pain of arthritis. These are the prostaglandins that occur as a result of disease. Newer NSAIDs selectively inhibit COX-2 and not COX-1. This leaves the housekeeping and protective mechanisms of "good" prostaglandins alone. These COX-2 selective inhibitors are COX-1 sparing and should not be associated with stomach ulcers and many of the other side effects of NSAIDs.

H. pylori infection is not a risk factor for NSAID-induced ulcer disease. If taking NSAIDs, an ulcer may or may not be NSAID-induced or secondary from *H. pylori* infection. Because the two types of ulcers are unrelated, treatment for one type won't help the other type. Everyone with proven stomach ulcers should be tested for *H. pylori* infection and if infection is present, treated with antibiotics.

Symptoms

Early symptoms of ulcer disease include nausea, heartburn, and stomach pain. Later, symptoms result from bleeding. Vomited blood looks like used coffee grounds, rather than bright red blood, and results in black tarry stools, lightheadedness, and faintness. Bleeding is a serious complication of stomach ulcers and should not be ignored. If symptoms like these occur while taking NSAIDs, this should cause concern and you should seek medical advice immediately. Researchers estimate in the United States each year there are thousands of deaths that occur as a result of bleeding ulcers or perforation of the stomach secondary to NSAIDs.

Fifty percent of ulcers induced by NSAIDs may be asymptomatic and cause no pain. An ulcer can bleed and perforate the stomach wall precipitating a life-threatening situation without any warning at all.

Though several approaches attempt to allow NSAIDs to be more tolerable, this doesn't necessarily make NSAIDs safer. This includes: taking medication with food, taking the medication in an upright position, or following the medicine with water. There is concern by some physicians that covering up NSAID symptoms with other medications is dangerous and puts you at an increased risk for bleeding.

Treatment

When the inflammation of arthritis is serious and requires continued treatment with anti-inflammatories, and there is a prior history of stomach symptoms or ulcer disease, several treatments can be tried before discontinuing NSAIDs. The drug misoprostol (Cytotec) is a synthetic prostaglandin that replenishes the naturally occurring "good" prostaglandins in the stomach wall. Patients taking misoprostol with NSAIDs experience far fewer stomach ulcers than those not taking the medication. Side effects of misoprostol are generally mild and include diarrhea and abdominal pain that usually subsides after a few days of therapy. Combination medications of NSAID with diclofenac and misoprostol (Arthrotec 50 or 75) are available. These medications add to the expense of taking NSAIDs. Nonacetylated salicylates like salsalate (Disalcid) or magnesium salicylate (Trilisate) do not induce ulcers as often as other anti-inflammatories, but are still considered ulcerogenic. Several enteric NSAIDs are coated tablets and have no direct effect on the stomach's lining, since they are absorbed farther down the GI tract. This does not prevent the effects of prostaglandin inhibition that occurs in the blood. Food may have a small beneficial effect. Finally, antacids like Mylanta or Maalox, and H2-receptor blockers like ranitidine (Zantac), cimetidine (Tagamet), nizatidine (Axid), or famotidine (Pepcid) work by neutralizing the stomach's acid or inhibiting acid production. These drugs do not necessarily prevent NSAID-induced ulcers, but are effective in healing ulcers. Potent acid inhibitors include proton pump inhibitors (PPIs) like omeprazole (Prilosec), rabeprazole (Aciphex), esomeprazole (Nexium), pantoprazole (Protonix), or lansoprazole (Prevacid) and provide greater protection than the H2-receptor blockers. Since many stomach ulcers occur without symptoms, there is concern that acid-blocking drugs can mask early symptoms and lead to a false sense of security.

The best treatment for prevention of stomach ulcers as a result of NSAID use is to minimize the use of these medications and use alternative mild pain relievers when appropriate. Acetaminophen (Tylenol) is not ulcerogenic, however, it is a pain reliever and not an anti-inflammatory medication. There are other risk factors that increase the chance of developing ulcers and bleeding from NSAIDs too, including smoking, alcohol, coumadin, other significant illness, increasing age, and prior ulcer history.

Disability

Disability as a result of an arthritis burden is significant. Arthritis and musculoskeletal disorders are the most prevalent major health problems in America. Arthritis affects over thirty million people aged forty-five years and older. About half are over age sixty-five. These illnesses have a major impact on disability benefits, medical care, and their corresponding costs. Arthritis increases in prevalence with increasing age. It is more common in women than in men. As America grays, the impact of arthritis will become more important. Arthritis ranks significantly as a cause of long-term disability, medical visits, and prescription and nonprescription drug utilization. Arthritis also accounts for a large number of all hospitalizations. The direct costs of arthritis medical care are estimated in billions of dollars every year. Clearly, arthritis care burdens health care. The costs of unproven remedies also rival these amounts.

RA and OA are chronic illnesses lasting many years. Disability and pain accumulates slowly as joint destruction progresses. Most people with RA experience a lifetime of remissions and flares requiring ongoing medical supervision. The medical management of arthritis involves frequent monitoring. Fortunately, many therapeutic regimens can produce measurable benefits and may modify the disease course, actually slowing the progression over time.

Disability and Handicap

Disability is a major problem for people with arthritis. Arthritis is responsible for marked reductions in work status and income. Over fifty percent of people with RA lose their employment after the disease occurs. As a group, people with RA earn only fifty percent of the income expected for them based on age and educational level. On this basis, disability has been established as one of the greatest problems facing people with arthritis. There is often confusion about the terms *disability* and *handicap*, although both have well-defined definitions. Disability is any restriction or lack of ability to perform an activity considered normal for most people. Handicap is defined as a disadvantage for a given individual, resulting from an impairment or a disability. Handicaps limit or prevent the fulfillment of a role that is normal for most people. Many people with arthritis need handicap parking or other advantages

that are not necessary for the general population.

Arthritis is a challenging disease. Difficulty derives from the many uncertainties surrounding the illness. It is not unexpected that depression is one of the most vexing problems for arthritis patients. The profound impact that depression can have on disability is significant. Persons depressed display more disability.

Psychological factors may be better predictors of disability than conventional disease activity measures.

At any rate, prevention, early recognition, and treatment of psychological factors like depression are important in minimizing disability and the impact of RA or other forms of chronic arthritis on society and the individual with a specific rheumatic illness.

The Americans with Disabilities Act

The Americans with Disabilities Act (ADA) became law in 1990, and is responsible for many changes. It prohibits discrimination against people with disabilities in employment, transportation, public accommodations, telecommunications, and services provided by the state and local government. Millions of people with arthritis are among those who benefit from this law. Disability related to arthritis encompasses not only those who use wheelchairs or canes and crutches, but also those whose disease leads to severe fatigue, limitations of movement, pain, or loss of strength.

If an employer has fifteen or more employees, the employer cannot discriminate against qualified applicants and employees on the basis of disability. (An employee is anyone working twenty or more hours per week.)

CRITERIA DEFINING A DISABLED WORKER

- Physical or mental impairment that substantially limits a major life activity
- A record of such impairment
- Regarded as having such an impairment

A major life activity includes performing manual tasks, walking, sitting, concentrating, and interacting with others, regardless of whether these tasks are required as part of the workplace responsibilities.

The employer is obligated to supply a reasonable accommodation for a qualified applicant or employee unless it would impose an undue hardship. A reasonable accommodation may be a modification or adjustment to a job that allows a disabled person to work.

The law allows a tremendous degree of latitude, instead of listing specific disabilities and accommodations. Slight changes at the workplace, bathroom, or bus can make independent living possible for people who would otherwise lead limited lives or be dependent on others.

Functional Classification

It is not uncommon to classify arthritis patients based on their ability to perform *self-care* activities including dressing, feeding, bathing, grooming, and toileting. *Avocational* activities include recreational or leisure time activities, while *vocational* activities include work, school, or homemaking. Function becomes a measurement of disease activity, a determination of prognosis, and a tool to determine the need for other interventions, treatment, or benefits like disability. Deterioration from one class to another in terms of needs, dependency, or reliance on others is a poor sign.

FUNCTIONAL CLASSES
Class I • Able to perform usual activities of daily living without help. • Class I individuals are normal with regards to their activities and have no limitations.
Class II • Able to perform usual self-care and vocational activities, but limited in avocational activities. Most of my patients are in this class. • Class II individuals are experiencing some effects of their disease with regards to recreational interests.
Class III • Able to perform usual self-care activities, but limited in vocational and avocational activities. • Class III individuals use walkers or even wheelchairs.
Class IV • Limited in ability to perform usual self-care, vocational, and avocational activities. This level of function is serious, since many of these patients will be bed-ridden. Staying in bed results in increasing medical problems and complications. • Class IV individuals are dependent on others for many of their basic needs. These patients put tremendous demands on resources.

The Real Truth About Arthritis

Truths about your arthritis are not always easy to learn. Many concerns or facts are not always correct. The more you can read and learn about your arthritis, the greater the chance of getting accurate and useful information.

Weather and Pain

Hold off packing if you are thinking of moving because of your arthritis for a warmer or dryer climate. The way the weather and climate affects arthritis is complex. It may not be actual weather changes that affect arthritis or joints, but stress or demands put on you. Stress creates effects on how you react to pain. Studies of the effects of weather on people indicate that symptoms worsen when the barometric pressure or humidity changes. Although a warmer and drier climate feels better, there is no scientific evidence it will halt the disease. Some of the largest arthritis clinics are in the warmest places.

If you are considering a move to a warmer climate, try spending a vacation there first to assess how it affects your symptoms. Many people are better on vacation, when away from day-to-day stress. The disadvantages of being away from friends and family may outweigh the benefits of warmer weather.

After Menopause

When women reach menopause, the supply of female hormone dwindles resulting in a loss of the benefits to the bone and heart. These problems are of concern for older women. This is recognized by medical researchers. Newer diagnostic tests and medications are available for postmenopausal women.

Stress and You

Stress does not cause arthritis and eliminating it will not end the disease. However, the impact of stress is a negative one. Arthritis is made worse by reactions to stress. Reactions vary from individual to individual.

Overdoing It

Too much exercise can increase the pain of arthritis. Pain following exercise is a signal

to take it a little easier, however, being too sedentary leads to increased stiffness. There should be a balance between exercise and inactivity or rest. During a flare of arthritis, rest more, but when you feel better, stay active to avoid stiffness.

Use it or lose it.
Move a joint daily to maintain range of motion.

Good Advice

Pay attention to your arthritis. Re-examine activities that aggravate your arthritis. Allow enough time for activities. Do not overdo. Use your stronger joints to carry or lift. Use a shoulder purse, rather than a hand-held wallet, if your hands are swollen. Get organized and conserve energy. When feeling well, prepare large meals for freezing and saving for later.

Total Hip Replacement

Total hip replacement (THR) is one of the greatest success stories of modern medicine. In the more than twenty-five years since the procedure was first introduced to Americans, almost one million have been performed. Cementing techniques have improved and complications such as infection and mechanical loosening have decreased significantly, as have rates of revision. Americans undergo 120,000 THRs annually. THR is done in those people experiencing moderate to severe pain. Overall outcomes from THR are very good and getting better all the time. Newer techniques have shortened hospital stays and lessened complications.

Drugs Over the Counter

Several years ago, the Food and Drug Administration (FDA) approved a nonprescription strength of popular anti-inflammatory medication, previously only prescribed. Some of these medications have now ended up on both sides of the counter, by prescription in higher doses and OTC in lower doses. Others have moved exclusively to the OTC status. The trend appears unlikely to abate and the future of self-medication seems bright. The drug industry obviously supports these OTC switches with high hopes.

When prescription medications go OTC, they are much more available. Since consumers need not see a physician or pharmacist, their use goes up quickly. In the crusade against rising health-care costs, self-medication represents one of the least costly components of health-care expenditures. Many consumers' insurance plans cover prescription medications but not OTCs. This results in more out-of-pocket expense for the patient. The fact that the OTCs cost less and are more available saves health insurance dollars and keeps health insurance premiums lower for the consumer.

One significant risk of OTCs is utilizing these medications for seemingly minor symptoms that are really signs of more serious diseases. As a precaution, the FDA has typically recommended lower dosages and label warnings about side effects and symptoms.

Liver Biopsy in Methotrexate Patients

Liver biopsy remains the gold standard for detection of cirrhosis, but the decision whether to perform a biopsy in MTX-treated RA patients is difficult for several reasons. The risk of developing MTX-induced cirrhosis is uncertain, the natural history of the liver disease is unknown, and there are no reliable clinical laboratory findings to guide the physician in the decision of when to perform a biopsy. With the increasing use of MTX as a long-term therapy in RA, this issue is of great importance. From the patient's standpoint, you must consider the risk of RA patients developing liver disease while receiving MTX, as well as the benefits, risks, and costs of performing a liver biopsy. In order to define the indications and timing of a liver biopsy in MTX-treated RA patients better, further research needs to focus on the incidence and natural history of this problem.

Collagen Vascular Diseases

Collagen is a substance made of protein that supports various structures throughout the body. It is the most important component of connective tissue found in blood vessels, skin, joints, kidneys, heart, and lung. Diseases affecting many of these organ systems are referred to as connective tissue diseases, or collagen vascular diseases. These same diseases are autoimmune and related to many forms of arthritis.

The First Few Months

Early diagnosis of different rheumatic diseases is difficult because of the similar clinical manifestations among several of the rheumatic diseases. A symmetrical arthritis of small- and medium-sized joints is the first symptom in rheumatoid arthritis, polymyositis, lupus, or scleroderma. On occasion, not until these disorders blossom into a definitive arthritis, is treatment programs and prognosis determined. Rheumatic illnesses can evolve into "overlap syndromes," appearing like more than one rheumatic illness or change characteristics to resemble a different connective tissue disease entirely.

Diet and More

Researchers have continually tried to determine how and why diet influences the course of arthritis. It is not clear to what extent foods affect the symptoms of arthritis. Eating a well-balanced diet to maintain energy and strength is as important for people with arthritis as it is for anyone else. Overweight people should lose weight to reduce the amount of stress on sore joints. Research has shown that only a small percent of people with arthritis flare after eating a specific food. If there is a specific food that does seem to aggravate arthritis, it should be avoided or eliminated from the diet. Currently, there is no special food that must be eliminated or added to the diets of people with arthritis.

Chondroprotective

Chondroprotective has been defined as an agent that can retard, arrest, or even reverse disease of human cartilage. It is suggested that some medications are chondroprotective, yet this remains to be proven. Unfortunately, this term is used in advertising and gives false impressions about the benefits of treatment that are not realistic at this time. No known treatment is currently chondroprotective.

Knuckle Cracking

Cracking your knuckles has no health benefits and causes no known long-term problems. The cracking sounds a joint makes when it is stretched, pushed, or pulled are caused by pressure within the joint capsule. Knuckle cracking does not lead to any type of arthritis or joint degeneration. Instead, it is an annoying habit.

Depression: Not Necessarily Part of the Disease

Depression occurs frequently during the course of arthritis. There is often uncertainty as to whether or not it is to be expected because of the stresses of the illness. States of depression are induced by the disease, by various medications used to treat arthritis, or by countless other factors in one's life. Depression is not to be confused with the everyday experiences of a mild mood swing that everyone experiences during difficulties. On the other hand, a serious depression is disabling, unpleasant, and prolonged. A variety of physical and psychological symptoms occur including sadness and gloom, crying without provocation, insomnia or restless sleep, loss of appetite or overeating, uneasiness or anxiety, irritability, feelings of guilt or remorse, lowered self-esteem, inability to concentrate, poor memory and recall, indecisiveness, lack of interest in things usually enjoyed, fatigue, and a variety of physical symptoms such as headache, palpitations, diminished sexual interest and/or performance, body aches, pain, indigestion, constipation, and diarrhea.

Just a few of these symptoms are enough to seriously disrupt life. Important symptoms are sense of failure, loss of social interest, sense of punishment, suicidal thoughts, dissatisfaction, indecision, and crying. People who feel hopeless believe that their distressing symptoms will never get better. People who feel helpless think they are beyond help and that no one cares enough to help them, or no one could succeed in helping them, even if they tried.

Many of the symptoms of depression go unrecognized in a chronic disease like arthritis. Symptoms are similar to those of the underlying medical condition. Even when recognized, depression goes untreated and/or inadequately treated.

The notion that those with chronic disease have a reason to feel depressed because they are sick should not be reinforced.

This interferes with early recognition, early treatment, and early relief of symptoms. Life with arthritis requires a series of adaptations and adjustments and each poses its own set of challenges. The need to develop new skills becomes important. It becomes necessary to focus on one success at a time, so that a pattern of success occurs more often than failure.

Survival

Studies in the long-term outcome of rheumatic diseases generally emphasize functional status, work disability, and the reduction of quality of life rather than survival or mortality. Yet, patients often ask their physician or family during the course of disease if they will die of their arthritis. The cause of death in individuals with rheumatic disease often is not recognized as rheumatic illness, but rather something more acute like stroke or heart disease. The more serious rheumatic diseases with higher death rates or mortality are rare, including SLE, vasculitis or scleroderma. Nonetheless, it is recognized that higher mortality rates are seen in arthritis and in most rheumatic illnesses than in the population without arthritis. Higher death rates are associated with more severe diseases. SLE with nephritis has one of the poorest responses of any disease. Death, unfortunately, should not be considered unrelated to arthritis. Rheumatic disease is considered a predisposing risk factor for infection, cardiovascular disease, or another condition to which death is attributed.

Osteoarthritis appears to be associated with higher death rates, although the rates are modest compared to the other inflammatory rheumatic illnesses like SLE. Even so, because OA is the most common rheumatic illness, higher mortality rates become an important health problem in the general population.

It is clearly understood now that patients with RA die at an age earlier than would be expected for individuals of the same age and sex in the general population.

RA is rarely mentioned on death certificates. RA is associated with a five-to-fifteen-year reduction of survival. There is a general underestimation of the mortality in RA. Patients with RA who are at risk of early mortality are identified by evidence of more severe systemic disease. Death is rarely explained by drug toxicity or other treatment as you might guess. SLE is associated with increased mortality rates. The past several years there has been significant improvement because of increased disease recognition, more sensitive diagnostic tests, as well as treatment. Early treatment appears to improve survival. Because of the predisposition to higher mortality rates among patients with rheumatic diseases, the argument is made that specialty medical care provided by a rheumatologist is both cost-effective and ethical in the long-term strategy for patients.

Managed Care

Health care is clearly in reform, and most of this has occurred without any specific laws passed. The anticipation of governmental involvement has resulted in significant changes in the delivery of health care in the United States. This impacts all those individuals with arthritis who rely on health care. Unfortunately, people with chronic illnesses have a continuous need for complex and expensive health care that makes them unattractive financial risks in the setting of managed care organizations (MCOs) and the capitation environment.

Managed care initiatives focus on controlling costs through gatekeeping provisions for subspecialist referrals. Medical subspecialties like rheumatology are potentially more affected by managed care systems because many arthritis problems are treated by the primary care physician. Gatekeeper restrictions about referrals potentially affect the arthritis patient's access to specialized rheumatology services.

It is possible that managed care organizations provide a well-managed system of care, however, there is limited evidence and information with regards to this now.

It may be that MCOs are not more efficient at delivering health care at a lower cost, but rather they provide less costly care, in part by providing lower quality care or less care.

In the field of arthritis, research is necessary to determine specific treatment protocols or algorithms utilizing allied health professionals trained in rheumatology in conjunction with primary care physicians and rheumatologists to form a new integrated health care provider organization. Much of this is well underway, but needs to be looked at with regards to final health care outcome.

Pregnancy

There is something very different about the immune system in pregnancy. Pregnancy alters the expression of the connective tissue diseases and results in some improvement or worsening of symptoms. There is no doubt that sex hormones influence the immune system. Most connective tissue diseases are more common in women than in men. Rheumatoid arthritis has a three-to-one ratio, women to men, and lupus nine to one. Lupus is much more common during the childbearing years. Medical reports suggest possible effects of lupus while some women take estrogen replacement therapy after menopause or hormones for contraceptive purposes earlier in life.

Many patients with rheumatoid arthritis experience relief of symptoms during their third trimester of pregnancy. Improvement with contraceptives or estrogens has led some alternative clinics to suggest this as treatment, even though this remains to be proven or accepted as standard therapy. During pregnancy, lupus patients improve, stay the same, or even worsen. Lupus patients have no difficulty getting pregnant; instead, the problem is staying pregnant and carrying a fetus to term safely. It is most important that the disease is quiescent at the time of contraception and that a pregnant women be off fetal-toxic drugs, especially antimalarials, and not expect to need them during pregnancy. Antiphospholipid antibodies are responsible for fetal loss, low birth weights, stillbirth, and miscarriage in lupus patients. These antibodies predispose to blood clots in the placenta. These same antibodies result in a false-positive test for syphilis. Other tests to monitor include the lupus anticoagulant, besides anticardiolipin antibodies. The neonatal lupus syndrome (NLS) allows maternal antibodies of pregnant lupus patients to cross the placenta. This results in transient rashes to the infant or more importantly complete heart block. The presence of the Ro antibodies (SS-A) in the mother predicts heart block in the newborn and alerts the physician. It is not a reason to terminate a pregnancy early, but knowing the antibody is present and the potential for heart block in the newborn allows for close monitoring of the fetus throughout pregnancy and the baby at the time of birth.Pregnancy is a special challenge in those individuals with connective tissue diseases.

Pregnancy is not to be avoided, but planned.

Timing and the control of the underlying disease and its manifestations are crucial. There are only a few patients who should avoid pregnancy entirely. These decisions can be determined in conjunction with a rheumatologist and experienced obstetrician.

Sexuality and Arthritis Go Together

While physicians are adequately prepared to help patients cope with different lifestyles because of arthritis, adjust to activities of daily living because of their disabilities, and deal with the domestic and marital problems brought on by the arthritis, few are trained for or feel comfortable discussing patient's sexual problems. The Arthritis Foundation (AF) has addressed this to some degree in a small booklet. Sexuality is very much a part of living and merits recognition and resolution; unfortunately, this subject often precipitates uneasiness during discussion. Many arthritis sufferers are older and are taught that sex is for the young. However, sexuality and sexual performance improves with age and experience.

Not only is sex important for the physical rewards, it is therapeutic for other reasons. The intimacy of sex also allows uninhibited communication, releases tension, and improves self-image.

For those individuals with severe arthritis, some helpful measures improve frequency, performance, and success. Planning in advance for sex includes setting the mood, observing the right time of day, or taking medicines to relieve pain. Communication makes it all happen. Comfortable positions help if a knee or hip problem is present and can be benefited by careful positioning or pillows.

Regardless of the obstacles, loving partners can adjust to each other and make sex possible just as it was before arthritis.

Bursitis and Tendinitis

Bursitis is inflammation of the small fluid-filled sacs that cushion areas adjacent to muscles or tendons moving over bones or other muscles. Bursa fluid prevents friction and protects the muscles and tendons from coming into direct contact with bones. Tendinitis results as a consequence of irritation of the tendon or cord that attaches muscle to bone near the joint. When a bursa or tendon becomes inflamed, there is pain and swelling in the localized area. There are over 150 bursae in the body, but the most commonly affected are the shoulders, elbows, hips, knees, and feet. Since bursitis or tendinitis mimics the same symptoms as arthritis, it is easily confused with arthritis. The inflammation is limited to surrounding tissues about the joint, rather than the joint itself. It tends to be very localized. Bursitis or tendinitis is not a chronic condition and most cases are self-limited. Bursitis or tendinitis resolves over a short period of time, although reoccurrences are common. The inflammation starts suddenly, lasts a few days or weeks, and subsides without any permanent damage.

Bursitis or tendinitis is caused by excessive pressure or incidental injury, but in most cases results from joint overuse or repetitive microtrauma. Repetitive microtrauma occurs while doing the same activity or motion over and over, sometimes hundreds of times an hour or day. Bursitis and tendinitis results because of a strain, overuse in athletic events, ill-fitting shoes, or excessive activities in people already deconditioned. Older people with arthritis are actually more prone to bursitis than younger conditioned individuals. Improper body mechanics irritate the bursa.

The primary symptom of bursitis or tendinitis is pain in the affected area. The pain is dull, persistent and increases with movement. It is disturbing at night and localized. If the bursa is swollen and hot, infection must be considered. Gout can occur in a bursa.

Bursitis or tendinitis is not discovered on an x-ray unless an occasional tendon calcifies. A physical exam by the doctor will confirm the diagnosis. Fluid can be drained from the localized area for examination and help determine if there is infection or crystals of gout.

Treatment and Prevention

Mild bursitis or tendinitis is initially treated at home with rest, elevation or icing, and over-the-counter anti-inflammatories. If the pain is severe or disabling, or doesn't subside spontaneously over a few days, consultation with a physician is necessary. Aspiration of fluid and injection with cortisone relieves pain quickly. Prescription doses of NSAIDs provide relief immediately. Rarely is surgery necessary in a troublesome bursa or tendon. Maintaining a full range of motion of the closest joint is important until the pain and inflammation resolves, so as not to lose range of motion permanently.

To prevent bursitis or tendinitis avoid activities that require repetitive motions. Repetitive activities result in microtrauma and should be avoided. Modifying work or play activities is helpful. Conditioning makes a significant difference. If pain occurs, a particular activity should be discontinued. Some athletic activities require additional instructions. Intermittent rest periods, changing grips on sport racquets, avoiding prolonged overhead activities, avoiding leaning on elbows, kneepads, safe lifting techniques, weight loss, good posture, regular exercise, and properly fitting shoes are all beneficial. Kneeling in the garden requires a cushion. Being aware of potential problems and performing regular range of motion exercises prevents many of the complications.

Hip Bursitis

Bursitis of the hip is common. Hip bursitis is uncomfortable when lying in bed, and painful when rolling from side to side. A localized area of tenderness to palpation occurs just over the bony prominence at the spot where the hand rests when standing erect and hangs down to the side. Anti-inflammatories or a local steroid injection provides pain relief. X-rays rarely show any changes from normal.

Elbow Tendinitis/Bursitis

Tendinitis occurs at the muscle attachment to the outside or inside of the elbow joint and is called tennis or golfer's elbow. Tendinitis after tennis and other sports, gardening, or carrying heavy objects is common at the elbow.

Bursitis results in swelling at the elbow and can occur in conjunction with rheumatoid arthritis, gout, infection or trauma. Bursitis at the elbow can swell as large as a golf ball or bigger.

Shoulder Tendinitis/Bursitis

A tear or inflammation of one of the muscles of the rotator cuff is common. The rotator cuff is a group of muscles surrounding the shoulder joint. Severe pain, aching, or pain with lifting the shoulder overhead is the first sign. Rotator cuff tears are easily visualized by x-ray procedures. A local steroid injection or anti-inflammatories helps transiently. Tears of the rotator cuff are degenerative and do not heal on their own. Surgical repair is necessary if simple measures do not first provide some relief.

Subacromial bursitis occurs close to the same area and produces similar symptoms. Bicipital tendinitis results in more pain in front of the shoulder. The pain prevents a full range of motion of the shoulder. A frozen shoulder or adhesive capsulitis occurs if all motion is lost and restricted secondary to pain. Range of motion exercises must be continued twice a day until the acuteness resolves. If adhesive capsulitis occurs and shoulder range of motion lost, it occurs over just a few days, but takes weeks to resolve or return to normal. Restricted motion of the shoulder makes it difficult to comb or brush the back of the head, put on coats or shirts, or put your hand in the back pocket of trousers. Some patients require a general anesthetic and then surgical manipulation of the shoulder to force motion and break up the adhesions about the shoulder that cause the restricted motion. Surgical manipulation can be associated with a fracture of the arm and is done only when other therapies fail.

Knee Bursitis

The anserine bursa is located just below the knee and on the inside of the leg. Pain in this area is easily confused with joint pain from the knee, although bursitis is usually well localized. Prepatellar bursitis is located just beneath the skin in front of the kneecap or patella and is very painful and swollen. Prepatellar bursitis is precipitated or aggravated by kneeling on the knee.

Foot Tendinitis

Achilles tendinitis occurs at the attachment of your calf muscle to the heel. This is a large tendon and becomes inflamed in some arthritic conditions or as a result of injury during sports. The tendon can suddenly snap and rupture making it impossible to push off with the toes of your foot. Surgery is usually required.

Pain occurs in several areas of the foot, especially the heel. Plantar fasciitis symptoms are common after inactivity or upon rising in the morning. The first several steps in the morning are very tender. Heel pain of plantar fasciitis can become severely disabling. Orthotics provide extra arch support, stretching relieves tightening, and weight loss unloads extra strains from the area. Local steroid injections, oral NSAIDs, or icing are beneficial. With time this will most often subside.

Hand and Wrist Tendinitis

Thickening or nodule formation on the tendons of the fingers results in pain, triggering, or locking. The nodule catches on the sheath that surrounds the tendon. Any finger can be involved. When a painful snap with motion occurs it is called a trigger finger. Rubbing the area is tender. Changing those activities that cause repetitive trauma or rubbing helps. Local steroid injections are useful, and on occasion surgery is required.

Extreme thickening and shortening of the fourth flexor tendon in the palm causes one or more fingers, especially the fourth, to bend towards the palm permanently, and is called Dupuytren's contracture. Surgery is sometimes required.

A painful form of tendinitis, called DeQuervain's tenosynovitis, results from overuse or inflammation of the tendons to the thumb and results in pain just above the wrist. This will prevent use of the hand during the simple activities like lifting a cup. Many of these people seek surgery for relief.

Drug Treatment of Rheumatoid Arthritis

Polypharmacy characterizes the drug treatment of rheumatoid arthritis (RA). It is rapidly changing over the years and deserves special mention in comparison to the drug treatment of other forms of arthritis. The drug treatment of RA can slow the course of disease as compared to the drug treatment of OA. Treatment was once based on a series of building blocks that slowly tapered and diminished in size so as to form a pyramid of treatment. At the base were more simple modalities like aspirin. As the pyramid went higher the selections were fewer in number, but much more potent and with potential for greater side effects. Historically, treatment has been polypharmacy, that is, several drugs in combination. This requires meticulous attention to possible drug interaction.

"Treating rheumatoid arthritis involves the subtle balance of suppressing disease while avoid-

ing side effects of medication. The goals of treatment are to decrease pain, improve function, and prevent joint damage. Patient education is the most important aspect of any treatment plan, as the development of coping mechanisms and realistic expectations allow for an improved quality of life."

Michael Charney, M.D.
Denver Arthritis Clinic
Denver, Colorado

The rheumatologist is the subspecialist of medicine possessing the expertise in the use of these different medications. Perhaps more than in any other field of medicine, the evaluation and treatment of RA is a true exercise in the art of medicine and good judgment. Experience has shown that the treatment of RA must be aggressive. Potent medicines must be used early in the disease course and in those individuals with poor prognostic signs. Recently, there has been a trend to invert the pyramid of treatment. Studies show that patients with active disease and other predictors of a poor prognosis develop joint damage or erosions of bones near the joint early within two years of onset of disease. Poor prognostic factors include an increased number of joints affected or a positive rheumatoid factor that is found in the blood of seventy-five percent of patients with RA. Most rheumatologists favor early aggressive treatment for these people.

There is no magical pill in the treatment of any form of arthritis.

Some of the oldest methods of arthritis treatment are now being questioned. Scientific studies done with medication for the treatment of RA must be interpreted carefully for both efficacy and risk. Efficacy includes the benefits and risks include real or potential side effects. If a medication does have side effects, it is hoped that problems as a result of side effects are not as severe as the disease itself. If the side effects are severe, then the medicine should be discontinued or kept to a minimum.

The drugs used in the management of RA can be divided into four different categories: miscellaneous medications, analgesics for pain, anti-inflammatory agents, and remittive drug therapy or disease-modifying antirheumatic drugs, DMARDs. It is important to know something about each group and how these medications work in concert.

Miscellaneous Medications

Miscellaneous medications include several different drugs, but are not limited to estrogen replacement therapy for postmenopausal women, antibiotics for infections, antihypertensives for the treatment of high blood pressure, cholesterol lowering agents, or perhaps something simpler like an over-the-counter vitamin or calcium tablets. Drug interactions need to be carefully considered.

POLYPHARMACY OF RHEUMATOID ARTHRITIS
MEDICATIONS

MISCELLANEOUS	ANALGESICS	ANTI-INFLAMMATORIES	REMITTIVE AGENTS
Hormones Antibiotics Supplements Birth Control Blood Pressure Etc.	Acetaminophen Narcotics Tylenol #3 Hydrocodone Tramadol	Salicylates or Aspirin Traditional NSAIDs NSAIDs (COX-2 Drugs) Oral Steroids Injectable Steroids	Antimalarials Gold Therapy D-penicillamine Imuran Methotrexate Arava Enbrel Remicade Cyclosporine Prosorba Column
Nothing to do with the Arthritis!	**Keep it Simple!**	**Symptomatic Treatment Only!**	**Slows the Progress of the Disease!**
Necessary for Good Health	Skip Powerful Narcotics! Demeral Percodan Talwin	Watch for Side Effects!	Disease-Modifying Antirheumatic Agents

Patients with RA are at special risk for stomach ulcers, infection, kidney problems and osteoporosis. Other problems should not be ignored. Since most patients are women, there may be special needs around the time of menopause including calcium and vitamin supplementation. The years of potential childbearing require effective contraception.

Drug regimens need modification during pregnancy or breastfeeding. Many acid-blocking drugs like nizatidine (Axid), famotidine (Pepcid), cimetidine (Tagamet), or ranitidine (Zantac) are available over the counter. More potent acid-blocking medications like rabeprazole (Aciphex), pantoprazole (Protonix), omeprazole (Prilosec) or lansoprazole (Prevacid) require a prescription. Misoprostol (Cytotec) replenishes prostaglandins which play a key role in inflammation, but a protective role for the stomach lining in the body's defense against its own acid. Newer drugs like selective COX-2 inhibitors rofecoxib (Vioxx), celecoxib (Celebrex), and meloxicam (Mobic) are important because of increased safety. It is impossible to list all miscellaneous medications.

Pain Medications

Analgesics are pain medications. They include narcotics. These medications are important, but perhaps require the greatest precautions and judicious use. Pain relievers mask pain without actually changing the arthritis. While treating a chronic incurable disease like RA with narcotic analgesics, there is always the possibility of developing dependence or even addiction for pain medications. Narcotics need not be avoided, but should be kept to the lowest possible dose that does the job. Narcotics commonly cause nausea, drowsiness, or constipation. Codeine derivatives especially cause these symptoms. There are some narcotic medications that have a greater predilection for abuse and should probably be avoided if possible, including oxycodone and aspirin (Percodan), or oxycodone and acetaminophen (Percocet), pentazocine (Talwin), meperidine (Demeral), or hydromorphone (Dilaudid). The use of these medications must be individualized to the needs of the patient.

*With regards to narcotics,
the rule of thumb should be,
"More is not always better."*

Some narcotics in small doses are acceptable and cannot be avoided, including propoxyphene (Darvon) or propoxyphene with acetaminophen (Darvocet N-100), codeine derivatives like hydrocodone (Vicodin), codeine with acetaminophen (Tylenol #3), or tramadol (Ultram). These medications are intended for people with moderate-to-moderately-severe pain.

Anti-Inflammatory Agents

Anti-inflammatory agents include several medications like aspirin (salicylates) or other aspirin-like medicines, nonsteroidal anti-inflammatory drugs (NSAIDs), or corticosteroids (steroids). Typically, these medications are not combined because of the added risk for side effects. Combining NSAIDs results in additive adverse events or the potential for "double trouble." This is rarely worth the risk.

*Anti-inflammatories do not change the
course of RA, but are symptomatic treatment only.*

Anti-inflammatories provide relief of symptoms like redness, swelling, warmth, and pain. In low doses, all of the nonsteroidal anti-inflammatories are pain relievers. They are prompt in onset so that relief occurs in minutes to hours. The reduction of the signs of inflammation takes several days. Most people believe there are no significant differences among all the available NSAIDs with regard to efficacy. There are some differences in the incidence of side effects and dose. Aspirin levels can be measured in the blood to determine adequate dosing and compliance. To reduce upset stomach, NSAIDs are taken with food, rather than on an empty stomach. Patients demonstrating intolerance to this group of drugs require a concomitant gastrointestinal (GI) protective agent. Unfortunately, many patients with serious GI side effects from NSAIDs never develop noticeable symptoms. There is concern that the concomitant use of antacids or acid-blocking drugs will cover up the symptoms of an ulcer and increase the risk for GI bleeding secondary to NSAIDs. Steroids are the most potent anti-inflammatory, but usually result in side effects that are not always acceptable.

Remittive Drug Therapy

Long-acting antirheumatic drugs have the potential to slow the progression of the disease. They are not a cure. These medications are considered disease-modifying antirheumatic drugs called DMARDs, second-line medications, or slow-acting antirheumatic drugs. DMARDs include gold or chrysotherapy (Solganol, Aurolate), d-penicillamine (Depen, Cuprimine) not related to the antibiotic, antimalarials like hydroxychloro-quine (Plaquenil) or quinacrine (Atabrine), sulfasalazine (Azulfidine) and immunosuppressive, chemotherapeutic, or anticancer drugs like methotrexate (Rheumatrex) or azathioprine (Imuran). Drugs suppressing rejection in organ transplantation are used, and include cyclosporine (Neoral, Sandimmune). Newer medications include leflunomide (Arava), entanercept (Enbrel), and infliximab (Remicade). The immunoadsorption column (Prosorba column) was approved by the FDA for the treatment of moderate-to-severe adult rheumatoid arthritis in patients with longstanding disease who have failed or are intolerant of DMARDs. The column binds a silica matrix to a protein that has the affinity to bind antibodies related to rheumatoid arthritis. The standard course of treatment is twelve weekly outpatient sessions.

There are a number of experimental medications currently undergoing research and new approaches to the therapy of RA on the horizon. New approaches are important to patients who develop refractory RA, in which the disease fails to respond adequately to prescribed treatments and runs a resistant course with progressive joint damage, deformity, and complications. The lack of a cure for RA and the inability to induce remissions with current drugs has led to the idea of combining DMARDs. These combinations are effective therapy.

The goal of drug treatment in RA is to induce a complete remission.

Interpreting Remission

There are many ways to interpret improvement or remission of RA in response to medicine. An accurate definition is more important in academic medicine or the comparison of different medications and their respective clinical efficacies. Physicians use a multitude of clinical and laboratory signs and symptoms during therapeutic decision-making in the management of RA. There is probably no right or wrong answer. It appears now that most available medications only achieve a remission while they are taken. Long-lasting remissions are unusual. Even so, a complete remission remains the goal of RA treatment. There is an occasional patient who goes into a spontaneous remission regardless of interventions. In older individuals with longstanding disease a remission is sometimes referred to as "burned-out RA." However, many rheumatic illnesses are characterized by good and bad times, peaks or valleys, which are not necessarily true and permanent remissions. These periods last days, weeks, or months. At the onset of disease an individual needs to be given a period of a few weeks to determine whether a spontaneous remission will occur without the need for drug therapy.

Outcome Measures of Remission

A set of outcome measures for the clinical trials of new treatment regimes has been developed by the American College of Rheumatology (ACR), and serves as another useful means with which to measure improvement or response to treatment.

MEASUREMENTS OF IMPROVEMENT IN RHEUMATOID ARTHRITIS
• Morning stiffness less than fifteen minutes
• No fatigue
• No joint pain
• No swelling
• Normal sedimentation rate

Other findings that may be followed include constitutional symptoms like fatigue, weight loss, or fever. An assessment of functional status or a measure of overall assessment by the physician or patient is also an important criterion to measure activity of disease and the need or response to treatment. Extra-articular manifestations of RA significantly affect prognosis and the severity of disease, and ultimately the institution and extent of treatment; thus their improvement suggests control of the inflammation of the disease. Extra-articular manifestations include anemia (a low red blood count), nodules (bumps at the elbows), a positive rheumatoid factor (a blood test marker for RA), and other organ involvement outside the musculoskeletal system.

Some patients will do well with one form of remittive therapy, and not another. Unfortunately, there is no way to predict who will do well with what, or who will develop a problem. Unfortunately, there is no simple blood test that will predict a response or a side effect to medicine. Remittive therapy needs to be initiated and monitored by someone experienced, usually a rheumatologist.

Principles of Remission

Regardless of the best definition of remission, there are several important principles:

- A reduced erythrocyte sedimentation rate (ESR) after treatment (if initially elevated) indicates less inflammation, and perhaps a response to treatment. This is a simple and relatively inexpensive blood test that has been utilized in medicine for over seventy years. Laboratories tend to use several different methods for this test, although the Westergren method is preferred by most experts in the treatment of arthritis. The ESR remains convenient, continues to be inexpensive, and enjoys familiarity with most physicians. However, it remains nonspecific and is elevated in other inflammatory states like infection, malignancy, or other rheumatic illnesses. The C-reactive protein (CRP) is another indicator of inflammation, and is more sensitive than the ESR. The CRP may also have some importance in monitoring the actual disease process, since it may indicate an interruption in the inflammatory process. These two laboratory tests are nonspecific indicators of inflammation and unfortunately fail to help differentiate RA from other forms of arthritis or other rheumatic illnesses. The major use of these tests is to monitor the clinical disease activity in patients with RA. Persistent elevations of these tests correlate positively with joint destruction. Improvement of these tests is objective evidence of a beneficial response to treatment. The rheumatoid factor is not significantly affected by treatment to have a value in monitoring response, even though it may go down slightly.

- A reduced need for anti-inflammatory medications suggests a response to treatment. Decreasing steroids just a few milligrams on a daily basis is important and a big step. Less nonsteroidal anti-inflammatories or pain medications is important. Effective treatment with NSAIDs is usually not associated with a significant change in the ESR.

- The patient's subjective interpretation of improvement includes less pain and less morning stiffness, a nonspecific subjective complaint of localized or generalized reduced mobility of the joints upon arising in the morning. This may be quantitated in minutes, hours, or may last all day, and usually suggests worse disease activity. This indicates less synovitis or actual inflammation around the joints.

- The physician's assessment of persistent arthritis is much like the patient's view, although usually more objective, and includes counting the number of swollen or tender joints and determining the duration of morning stiffness.

- Finally, any definition or criterion for remission includes an improved quality of life. This becomes an essential part of treatment, and coincides with the relief of pain and improved function. Even individuals with impairments that result in loss of function with activities of daily living, work, or recreation can still desire and attain an improved quality of life. Besides the dimensions of physical limitations, social and emotional aspects become increasingly important. It is possible that some treatment regimes of RA work exceedingly well, yet result in social and emotional problems that ultimately outweigh any gains.

In most cases, a complete remission is not achieved. The management of RA then is to control the progression of disease activity, alleviate pain, maintain activities of daily living, maximize quality of life, and slow the rate of joint damage.

Surgery

Surgery plays a role in those individuals experiencing unacceptable pain and/or limitation of function due to structural joint damage. Whether inflammation of the joints is successfully controlled or eliminated, patients may have already experienced significant joint damage. The most successful surgical procedures include carpal tunnel release at the wrist, resection of the heads of the metatarsal bones of the foot near the toes, joint replacement of the large knuckles of the hand, and total hip and total knee replacements. For most patients with arthritis, surgery will never be necessary. Their arthritis is controlled with conservative management like medications, physical or occupational therapy, exercise, and rest.

Recent advances in the field of orthopedics within the past several years has made a significant impact on improving the quality of life of patients with arthritis more than has progress in any other area of arthritis. Unfortunately, the course of most arthritis is persistence and drug therapies vary in their effectiveness. Therefore, many of the patients with chronic forms of arthritis will develop structural damage that requires surgical intervention. It is unusual to have all the joints involved at the same time, usually only a few joints are involved at a time. It is these joints that will probably suffer the most damage. The structural damage that does occur is usually irreversible and additive, that is, only worsening over time. The patient becomes more symptomatic and has increasing difficulties with functional activities. This argues for early aggressive medical management of the disease and options of surgical interventions later in the disease, when structural damage becomes the dominant factor. In addition, consideration must be given to operating on one or a few joints in a disease that affects many at one time. The question must be asked whether the stress of surgery and the postoperative period is worth the results. This is difficult to decide. The decision to have surgery is a serious one, and should never be taken lightly. You need to be well informed, educated, and aware of other options or alternative treatments, including not having surgery. Second opinions from other surgeons are reasonable if the second surgeon is provided all the available medical records, x-rays, laboratory tests, and is also allowed to reexamine the patient.

Orthopedic Surgeon

The rheumatologist will often have several surgeons as referral sources. Friends and family know orthopedic surgeons who have cared for them or loved ones. Previous experience and trust with a known surgeon helps establish a good doctor–patient relationship during a difficult time. However, the surgeon must have experience with arthritis, besides being capable of relating to the patient, family, and rheumatologist.

It is important that the patient and family have realistic expectations about the outcome of the surgery, both in respect to appearance and function, but also potential complications and postsurgical needs including physical therapy, extra help at home, and medications, especially for pain control.

The rheumatologist should orchestrate the timing of surgery in patients with rheumatoid arthritis because of the complexity of the issues.

It is not uncommon that individuals with rheumatoid arthritis will need several surgeries. Prior to surgery, there are special needs for medication changes, including extra steroids if the patient has already taken steroids for a prolonged period of time or eliminating medications that aggravate bleeding.

Indications for Surgery

Evaluating the need for surgery is difficult, although the primary indications are either improved function or relief of pain. To operate for pain relief alone is sometimes a difficult decision, however, pain at night or nocturnal pain is often a clear-cut indication for joint replacement in hip disease.

SURGICAL INTERVENTION CATEGORIES IN ARTHRITIS

- Arthroscopy (looking with a scope)
- Arthrotomy (opening the joint)
- Synovectomy (removing the lining of the joints)
- Resection (removing the joint)
- Arthrodesis (fusing the joint)
- Replacement (artificial joints)

- *Arthroscopy* is looking into a joint with a small scope. The scope contains a camera and passages to allow instruments to enter into the joint. With eyes on the monitor, the surgeon moves instruments around within a joint to scan and look, retrieves material, and repairs torn structures. Originally used in large joints like the knee,

arthroscopies are now utilized in almost all joint spaces and other spaces within the body. Arthroscopy is not a first line of treatment, but becomes an important procedure and sometimes, final treatment for certain conditions. The procedure is typically done on an outpatient basis under a general anesthesia, or in many cases local or regional anesthesia. This allows a quick recovery and return to activities. During the procedure, small nicks of the skin allow the instrument with a camera to enter the joint space. A tube is inserted to allow the introduction of fluid into the joint. Large amounts of sterile fluid put into the joint enlarge the space and provide a better view; a second tube allows the fluid to escape and help flush the joint space of unwanted debris and inflammatory products within the joint space. Complications of arthroscopy are unusual, but may be related to the need for a tourniquet that prevents bleeding during the procedure, the introduction of foreign material into the joint, or the immobility required following the procedure. Other complications include blood clots, infection, bleeding into the joint, or even nerve damage. The advantages over opening the joint or *arthrotomy* are tremendous. The recovery period following arthroscopy is significantly shortened, walking and mobility occur much more quickly, and the costs are less compared to a prolonged stay in the hospital.

- *Synovectomies* are the removal of inflammatory tissues in and around the joint, including the sheath around tendons next to the joint. These procedures are done to prevent further damage to the tendons and joints. The ends of the bones (articular surfaces) are left intact and hopefully preserved. The popularity of synovectomy in recent years has declined compared to past years when the removal of the lining of the joint at surgery was more in favor. By removing the inflammatory tissues about the joint, it is felt that this prevents damage to the articular cartilage covering the ends of the bones. Regardless, this type of surgery is still appropriate on occasion and provides palliative relief for years in those individuals with disease limited to a just a few joints. The inflammatory tissues around a tendon are removed surgically for the relief of triggering or other dysfunction of the tendons. Sometimes as much can be achieved by locally injected steroids. Tendon rupture requires repair as well as removal of the inflammatory tissue.

- *Resection* arthroplasty removes a portion of an otherwise damaged joint. This procedure is done when the joint is not necessary for weight-bearing. Metatarsal-phalangeal (MTP) resection, the removal of the heads of the bones at the base of the toes is a good surgery and provides important relief to the patient with arthritis.

The arthritis causes these joints to become prominent. The patient feels as though they are walking on marbles. Removal of the head of the radius bone at the elbow is helpful for the movement of the hand.

- *Arthrodesis* or joint fusion alleviates pain within the joint at the sacrifice of motion. It should be avoided if possible, but in some cases there is no choice. Fusion of the end joint of the thumb is useful and allows improved function when instability of that joint interferes with a strong pinch of the thumb against the index finger.

- *Joint replacement* surgery or reconstructive procedures create a definite change in the joint, sometimes removing it entirely. Joint replacement is considered in those individuals when inflammation of the cartilage has destroyed the joint. This is seen on the x-ray as severe joint space narrowing and felt on physical examination as crepitation. Total joint replacement (THR) has revolutionized the care of patients with all forms of arthritis. Concern centers around the durability of the prosthesis. Although revision of total joints is difficult, it is certainly possible. Durability is limited because of possible loosening or the occurrence of infection. The major complication of total joint replacement is infection. Infection requires removal of the artificial joint and a prolonged period of immobility while the patient is functionally without a joint. Removal of an artificial hip still allows some ambulating around the house on crutches, while the removal of a knee joint limits one to transferring from bed to chair until antibiotics are finished and the artificial joint can be replaced. The evaluation of a painful artificial joint requires aspiration or removal of fluid with a needle placed through the skin surface to examine for infection.

Pain relief after total joint replacement is usually prompt, although there is obviously postoperative pain that must resolve over time. The replacement of the shoulder joint has unique obstacles for the patient and the surgeon. Patients with severe RA associated with destruction of the shoulder joint will invariably have significant deterioration of the rotator cuff, an important group of muscles around the shoulder joints. This often precedes advanced destruction of the articular cartilage. Shoulder muscles around the joint are also damaged and limited because of disuse. After shoulder replacement, the range of motion is not always as good as anticipated. This argues for seeking a shoulder joint replacement early.

Timing of Surgery
Except for a few instances, surgery in the arthritis patient is elective. There are few indications for emergency operations. Immediate intervention is necessary if there is evidence to suggest instability of the cervical spine, which could result in serious impingement or pressure on the spinal cord and nervous system function. Fusion of the first two cervical vertebras is not uncommon and the results are usually excellent. Rupture of a tendon may be an emergency. Surgery is necessary not only to repair the tendon, but also to prevent further damage. Finally, drainage of an infected joint or removal of an infected prosthesis is almost always an emergency surgery. While debating surgery for the arthritis patient, one must understand that orthopedic surgery is only one of several options to consider in an attempt to integrate the total management and care of the patient. Important principles include the understanding that the disease cannot be cut out by surgery alone, and to operate for pain alone usually results in more pain for the patient. Other complications occur as a result of concurrent medical problems, like coexisting heart disease. The required immobility increases the potential for pneumonia or blood clots to the lungs and the potential for hospital acquired disease or iatrogenic illness, including a blood transfusion or drug reaction.

Ask Questions about Surgery
If you're thinking about surgery, realize it involves a recovery period. Surgery has no guarantees. Remember, ask questions about the surgical procedure and recovery period.

Bloodless Surgery

It is not uncommon during joint replacement surgery that blood transfusions become necessary. Following major joint replacement like hip replacement, fewer blood transfusions are given now as compared to several years ago because of the concern for transmitting infection like hepatitis. Patients are allowed to build up their red blood cells screening and improvements to laboratory markers have reduced the risk for HIV and hepatitis C infection. Despite improvements, a zero-risk blood supply does not exist.

Bloodless medicine and surgery programs are established to meet the demands for medical and surgical treatment without the

---

QUESTIONS TO ASK THE SURGEON

- How will surgery improve function and decrease pain?
- How long will the operation take?
- How long will I be in the hospital, or can the operation be done as an outpatient?
- Will a blood transfusion be necessary or can I donate blood before surgery?
- Will I need any special equipment at home following surgery?
- Following surgery, will therapy be necessary?
- Following surgery, will special medication be necessary?
- Will my blood be thinned and put me at risk for bleeding?
- How soon can I return to my normal activities such as driving or work?
- Will surgery, medicines, monitoring, or therapy be covered by my health insurance plan?
- How soon after surgery will I need to go in and see the doctor?

---

themselves prior to their surgery by taking iron supplements. Autologous blood transfusions or self-directed transfusions are donated several days before elective surgery and given postoperatively as needed. On occasion though, transfusions are still necessary. The blood supply in the United States has never been safer. The risk for infection with transfusion-transmitted viruses has never been lower. Expansion of blood donor use of donor blood or stored blood (whether for religious or personal reasons). Objectives of various bloodless strategies are to utilize all available resources to minimize blood loss. Techniques include salvage and the re-infusion of as much of the patient's own blood as possible, various cell-salvage techniques at the time of surgery, and treatment with specific medications designed to maximize the patient's own blood production.

Methods of salvage and reinfusion of blood at the time of surgery include the suction and saving of blood that is then filtered and then reinfused as a blood transfusion into the vein. During operations associated with significant bleeding, this can save large amounts of blood. Newer surgical techniques result in less bleeding at the time of surgery. Many operations routinely done through large incisions in the past are now done with small scopes inserted through the skin. These methods limit bleeding and other complications. Finally, medications that stimulate the production of both red and white blood cells are readily available and allow blood counts to dip lower than previously acceptable during the postoperative period.

Physical and Occupational Therapies

Physical therapy and occupational therapy are two of several different allied health care professional groups who help the arthritis patient. Maintaining the function and productivity of patients with arthritis requires coordinated multidisciplinary care, that is, several health care professionals including nursing, physical and occupational therapists, social workers, dietitians, educators, psychologists, and rehabilitation specialists. At least two deserve special mention. Physical therapists can demonstrate exercises to keep bones and muscle fit and strong. Occupational therapists help with activities of daily living (ADLs), especially upper extremity activities, splints, or assistive devices that can make life easier or more accessible.

Exercise
Exercise can help maintain range-of-motion (ROM), strength, and endurance, as well as making further

gains and improvements. If joints and muscles hurt, exercise may be the last thing on your mind, however appropriate exercise is important and beneficial. The stronger the muscles and other tissues around a joint become the better they will be able to support and protect an inflamed joint. Without exercise, the joint only becomes stiff and less mobile and the muscles weaker. The most comfortable position for a painful joint is flexion (bent), but keeping the joints in this position, encourages them to stay this way and limits their ability to straighten entirely. Typically, bent joints are not as strong; a good example is your handgrip. When the wrist is extended (held up), it is actually stronger than when the wrist is flexed. Propping a swollen and painful knee up in bed in a flexed position with pillows should be discouraged, since this encourages the joint to stay this way. Walking around with bent knees is difficult, and actually requires more strength than normal walking. Range-of-motion exercises are most important at the shoulder, since there are few activities done regularly during the day to preserve a full range of motion. Simple shoulder exercises can be done in the shower with hot water hitting the painful area. More difficult shoulder exercises include a pendulum exercise, that is, bending at the wrist and hanging the arm down, while swinging a light weight in all directions like a pendulum, while the other arm and hand support you on a safe and sturdy table.

For people with arthritis an exercise program should be individualized and include range-of-motion, endurance, and strengthening exercises. All programs planned by therapists should eventually be for home or other independent programs, for example a community swimming program. It should not be the intention of a therapist to have patients return for extended periods of time, (most insurance will not pay for maintenance programs). To justify several therapy sessions, there must be continued progressive improvement and the need for close monitoring by a physical or occupational therapist.

By improving range-of-motion, endurance, and strengthening through exercise, day-to-day activities become easier, safer, and more enjoyable. Exercise improves overall health and fitness by increasing energy levels, sleep and rest, weight, cardiac reserve, building stronger bones and muscles, and improve mood, self-esteem, and sense of well-being. Exercise also prevents injury and even prevents further joint damage by making cartilage healthier. By improving the range of motion in the hip or knee, significant functional impairments are avoided. Getting up from a low chair is difficult if the knee is swollen or painful.

Isometric Exercise

There are two important types of strengthening exercises. Isometric exercises involve tightening the muscle, but not really moving the joint itself. This is especially helpful when actual movement of the joint hurts. This helps build strong muscles without precipitating pain that might discourage further activities. Isometric exercise helps stabilize joints and provide a more even distribution of weight to prevent further injury. The best examples of an isometric exercise are quad sets, in which you tighten the large muscles at the front of the thigh without bending the knee itself. These can be done in bed, but are even better sitting upright in a good supportive chair with the leg put out parallel to the floor and held up for a few seconds twenty or thirty times twice a day.

Isotonic Exercise

Isotonic exercises involve moving the joint, and build strong muscles by slowly increasing the number of repetitions or adding light weights. Pool therapy helps by adding resistance while adding benefit from the buoyancy and warmth of the water. The water supports the body, putting less stress on the larger joints, and the warm water relaxes the muscles. Warm water provides immediate relief and allows motion to occur. Several exercises can be done in a shallow area of a pool without swimming. Most communities have water programs and many are sponsored by the Arthritis Foundation (AF). Health clubs have a wealth of equipment that helps accomplish many of the same goals in an interesting and different way.

Endurance Exercise

Endurance exercises are beneficial to people even without arthritis. Active exercises increase energy, stamina, help control weight, and improves mood. Simple activities include walking, swimming, and biking. These exercises encourage individuals to reach specific goals, increase walking capacity, and improve daily activities. Muscle disuse from inactivity quickly erodes strength. Muscles atrophy or shrink to thirty percent in one week and when at complete rest three percent per day. Once a swollen knee improves, strengthening the quadriceps muscles can actually decrease pain and increase function.

Aerobic Exercise

Aerobic exercises involve repetitive activities of large muscles aimed at increasing cardiovascular efficiency and improving muscular endurance and activity tolerance. Patients with arthritis can successfully perform aerobic exercises without exacerbating the underlying signs and symptoms of arthritis. Walking groups can increase walking distances, function, and decrease arthritic pain levels in those individuals with arthritis of the knee. Aerobic activities should be specifically tailored to a patient's needs, begun slowly, and minimize symptom aggravation to maximize compliance. Common aerobic exercises include walking, stationary bicycle riding, and swimming. Since the buoyancy of the water unloads the joints, aquatic exercises are helpful for those individuals with pain on weight-bearing.

Exercise Precautions

An exercise program has to be approached with care to minimize risk.

EXERCISE PRECAUTIONS

- Consult a doctor or exercise specialist who can design a specific safe and effective program for your needs.
- Warm up slowly before any exercise to prevent injury.
- Exercise when the arthritis is best controlled, although an inflamed joint still needs range of motion if possible, and some strengthening if not worsened by movement.
- Exercise the whole body.
- Protect the joints with adaptive equipment or special handles on equipment, if necessary.
- Use good posture and strengthen weakened muscles.

Physical fitness and training declines with age; that decline is accelerated in those individuals with arthritis. Proper exercise training reverses or at least slows this process. Overloading the muscular system is known as resistance training or weight-training and is currently popular at health fitness centers. This kind of training results in improved muscular strength, endurance, and recovery from the stresses imposed by physical activity and injury. The maintenance of muscle mass has been demonstrated to be increasingly important in the reduction of body fat, improvement in cardiorespiratory fitness, reduction of blood pressure, and improved blood lipid (cholesterol) profiles. In those individuals with arthritis and related conditions, resistance training increases the potential for a greater quality of life.

Heat or Cold

Therapists will often use different thermal modalities to provide relief to a swollen and painful joint. Warmth provides a soothing and sometimes deep penetrating relief, but should be done carefully with close monitoring. Heat relaxes muscles and stimulates the circulation. Cold temperatures provide pain relief.

Two opposite modalities, heat or cold can temporarily relieve the pain and reduce the swelling of some forms of arthritis, yet neither method works for all people all the time. Some people prefer heat, while others prefer the cold, and some do not prefer either. Yet, others get relief by alternating heat and cold to an affected area. Finding the most effective treatment requires a certain amount of trial and error.

Heat and cold have distinct advantages compared to other modalities at the therapist's hands. Most heat and cold applications are readily available at home without any large expense. A package of frozen peas makes an excellent ice pack until it becomes too mushy. Electrical heating pads are readily available in most households. Except for falling asleep with too hot a heating pad, there are few side effects. Sleeping with a heating pad for a prolonged period is dangerous and should be avoided; it can burn and mottle the skin. A physician can prescribe heat or cold treatments with a therapist to help discomfort, inflammation, swelling, and stiffness, and to relax muscles to facilitate motion and exercise. Heat tends to stimulate the circulation in a localized area and cold tends to numb an area and reduce inflammation. For many people who have arthritis, a hot shower in the morning is all they need to loosen their stiff joints.

Heat or cold should be applied in short intervals, perhaps only 15 to 20 minutes at a time.

Superficial heating is provided by hot packs, hot showers or baths, rubs or even paraffin wax treatments. Hot packs are moist or dry, and can also include mud baths, spa water, or mineral baths.

Diathermy is a method of deep heating. Ultrasound is the deepest of all heating modalities. These treatments are usually given by a therapist or doctor.

Ice packs, cold baths and cool sprays of chemicals like ethyl chloride relieve pain for periods of time. When heat or cold is applied, it only penetrates a few millimeters below the skin, yet this has beneficial effects. Although short-lived, if applied during exercise periods, improved range of motion occurs and the benefits are more long lasting.

During the immediate period following an intra-articular steroid injection, it is best to use ice for any discomfort. This slows any chemical reaction or response to the injection materials.

A towel between the skin and heat source or cold protects the surface of the skin from injury. Extreme temperatures should never be used, and topical creams should be avoided at the same time. Heat or cold treatments are applied only to healthy, clean, and dry skin. Open sores or cuts should be protected and checked regularly for infection.

Transcutaneous Electrical Nerve Stimulation

Transcutaneous electrical nerve stimulation (TENS) is a means of pain control available without the use of medication. It offers pain relief using a tiny electrical impulse. It has been in use since the late 1960s. The body of the unit houses batteries and operating controls; electrodes are then attached with small wires to adhere to the skin and over the area of pain. The electrodes direct a small electrical charge to the spot that produces the most effective pain control. The unit is mobile and is easily carried. The spot can be changed from day to day for the most effective coverage of pain relief. It is believed that the tingling created by the electrical stimulation blocks the brain's ability to receive pain stimulation, almost like a telephone line that can handle only one message at a time. Others believe that the electrical stimulation by the small unit stimulates the brain to produce its own pain-killing chemicals. Two basic modes on the unit allow either a constant tingling sensation to block other pain signals, or a pulsating charge to stimulate the brain's production of its own natural painkillers.

The reaction to a TENS unit is quite variable and individualized. Some people will receive no benefit and others cannot function without them. Most patients will receive some pain relief, although the response may differ depending on the type of pain relief sought.

The success of TENS depends on the situation. One may have to experiment with the location of the electrodes, adjusting the mode of current, a steady charge or pulsatile one, and the intensity of the charge. An experienced physical therapist can help with regards to it use, especially during a period of evaluation.

Help at Home

Occasionally, the disability of arthritis at the hips, knees, or even ankles, makes it difficult to get into buildings elevated even by only one step. If one lives on the second story, without an elevator, the difficulties make it nearly impossible. Ramps provide an alternative to either elevated or lowered areas for people who cannot use stairs. The slope of a ramp is the most important consideration. The maximum slope of a ramp should be twelve inches of length for every inch of rise or less. The minimum width should be thirty-six inches. Low curbs or edges will prevent wheels of a wheelchair or walker from going off the sides of the ramp. Handrails are usually installed thirty-six inches above the ramp. Outdoor ramps need antiskid texture and must be built to avoid accumulation of water or ice.

Choosing a Cane

A cane is intended to offer some amount of weight support while walking. A single point cane is for those who need minimal degree of support and stability. A quad cane is for those individuals with limited mobility, but who need a more stable cane. A variety of handles are available on canes including a crook style, tee style, orthopedic style, or swan neck style. The handle helps to distribute the weight evenly for additional support and a comfortable grip. It is important that a cane is adjusted to the proper length. To find the proper length, stand as naturally as possible on a firm and flat surface. Wear day-to-day shoes that are also comfortable. Let your arm hang down naturally. The cane is the proper length when the handle of the can touches the inside of your wrist where it meets the palm. A cane must be adjusted to the proper height. Many adjustable canes are made of metal and have adjustable locking collars. Wooden canes require removing the rubber tip from the bottom and sawing off some of the tip to the correct length.

Occupational Therapy

Like the physical therapist, the occupational therapists (OTs) are important allied health-care professionals that deal with exercise, strengthening, range of motion, and joint protection. Joint protection lessens pain and

---

THERAPY RECOMMENDATIONS FOR ARTHRITIS

- Use **support devices** for walking.
- Use a **cane**, crutch or walker to help reduce strain on the hips and knees.
- Use an extra-thick pen when writing; this puts less stress on the finger joints.
- **Long-handled tools** and special reaching devices give better leverage while gardening, cleaning, or retrieving goods from the shelf in the kitchen.
- Use a **bookstand** to hold a book while reading; this will avoid neck strain from looking down.
- Arrange furniture in a room for **safety** and comfort.
- Avoid climbing stairs by moving a bedroom or bathroom to one floor.
- Install **handrails** by the toilet, bathtub, stairs or steps into the house for extra support. A raised toilet seat will make the bathroom easier and safer.
- Have a comfortable chair with a high seat cushion that makes getting up easier, armrests to help getting up, and a good firm **back support** for sitting.
- Bend your knees when lifting and keep your back straight.
- Slide forward on a chair to get up.
- Push off with your forearms, if necessary.
- Wear well-cushioned athletic shoes with **good support**.
- Avoid high heels.

---

discomfort associated with some activities and discourages deformity. There are some activities done during the day that actually increase the tendency toward deformity. Splinting an inflamed wrist at night lessens the symptoms of carpal tunnel syndrome or keeping the wrist partially extended provides for a stronger power grip. On occasion deformities are so severe that the OT manufactures a custom splint.

Activities of Daily Living

Occupational therapists help with activities of daily living (ADLs), especially upper extremity activities, splints, or assistive devices that make life easier or more accessible. With a bit of ingenuity and specialized training the OT finds less stressful ways for the patient to do almost any activity. Placing heavy objects on lower shelves in the kitchen, a grab bar by the toilet or a rail handle on the one step from the garage into the house can make a world of difference for some people. Planning in advance, resting periodically, carrying smaller and fewer loads, and utilizing handles on grocery bags are helpful. Other important devices or ideas include: elastic shoe laces, slip-on shoes, built up handles on pencils or eating utensils, Velcro instead of buttons, long-handled shoe horn, button hook, zippers with pull rings and more.

Work Simplification

Conserve energy and make it simple. Avoid prolonged sitting, standing, or pressure on the same joints for long periods. Slide rather than lift, keep heavy objects on the lowest shelf, use multipurpose and lightweight equipment with built up handles if necessary. This makes grasping easier and safer. Limit activities to a few minutes. Clean house over several days, rather than just one or two.

Joint Protection

Joint protection avoids forces and stresses that damage joints. The force of a joint depends on the amount of weight it has to support and the length of time the movement takes. If muscles exert too much force over an inflamed joint, the tissues around the joint no longer support it or keep the muscles aligned properly. For example, carry a purse or shopping bag on the shoulder, so as not to aggravate the hands and avoid putting pressure on the fingers that encourages ulnar deviation or movement away from the thumb. Whenever possible, use a stronger joint to protect a weaker one. Distribute the weight of an object evenly on extremities, push through the palms of your hands whenever possible, instead of a closed fist, and pressure on the back of the hand.

Steroids

Steroids are one of the most important discoveries of modern medicine. Since their introduction in 1949, the use of cortisone-like drugs, steroids, or corticosteroids in the management of rheumatic diseases has remained controversial. There are several different preparations of steroids. The steroids utilized in the treatment of arthritis are not the same as sex hormones in birth control pills, or the steroids used in body building to increase muscle mass (anabolic). In fact, cortisone-like drugs actually break down muscle (catabolic) and lead to weakness and small muscle mass. Prednisone and methylprednisolone (Medrol) are the most common oral preparations. They are relatively inexpensive. Steroids are taken orally, by injection (parenteral) into muscle or intravenously for more systemic effects. Systemic effects occur throughout the body and affect many organ systems. Steroids are injected directly into a painful swollen joint or an inflamed area like a bursitis or trigger point for a more localized effect. Preparations for soft tissues include triamcinolone (Kenalog) or methylprednisolone (Depomedrol). Even localized injections like these however, result in a systemic effect. Injecting the right knee with a steroid may result in some benefit to the left knee. A localized steroid injection may transiently aggravate the control of diabetes because of the systemic effect of steroid on glucose control. This is usually not serious.

It has been reported that long-term low-dose prednisone orally (usually at <10 mg/day) has been used in the treatment of approximately one-third of RA patients seen in clinical practice. Controversy exists whether there are benefits with regard to disease activity, functional capacity, or x-ray progression of the arthritis.

Side Effects

The major drawback of steroids is serious side effects. Because steroids are frequently used in the treatment of RA the delicate balance between efficacy and toxicity must be monitored. If steroids are used in high doses for prolonged periods, side effects are guaranteed. By keeping the dose relatively low in a disease like RA (a disease that is usually not life threatening), side effects are minimized in relationship to the benefits to be gained. Most doses of steroids useful in clinical practice, taken for long enough, will re-

sult in at least some side effects. Most of the side effects are reversible. Unfortunately, weight gain for example, like any other weight gain is difficult to shed. A vertebral spinal compression fracture because of steroid-induced osteoporosis is not reversible and leads to a severe painful back condition. Steroids should not be avoided because of a

STEROID PROBLEMS
• Obesity
• Osteoporosis
• Hypertension
• Facial hair
• Cataracts
• Unusual infections
• Depression
• Anxiety
• Mood swings
• Yeast infections
• Shingles
• Bruising
• Muscle weakness
• Muscle wasting
• Diabetes
• Thin skin
• Gastritis or ulcers
• Striae of the skin
• Blurred vision
• Acne

fear of side effects. Doses should always be kept to a minimum. Alternate day steroids avoid some side effects, although some disease states require daily dosing without changes from day to day to respond. If a medical problem is considered life-threatening or serious, high-dose steroids of 60 mg/day or more are required to achieve the therapeutic effect desired. In that situation, side effects will occur until the dose is safely tapered.

Hip Pain

A serious complication of steroid use in rheumatic diseases, especially in systemic lupus erythematosus (SLE) is an abnormality of the hip. The hip is a ball and socket joint that is weight-bearing. The circulation of the ball portion of the hip becomes compromised and the bone dies (avascular necrosis). This results in collapse and serious disruption of the joint. This may occur in other or multiple joints and require surgery, including joint replacement.

Adrenal Suppression

An adrenal gland sits just above each kidney and produces cortisol equivalent to about 5 mg of prednisone daily. Cortisol maintains normal physiological functions of the body including blood pressure, fluids, and the balance of electrolytes like sodium and potassium in the blood. It is safe to take medical doses of steroids on occasion for periods of less than two weeks without significant suppression of the adrenal glands and their ability to make cortisol. Steroids taken for long periods of time result in suppression of the adrenal glands and their ability to produce cortisol for normal functions.

After oral steroids are taken for prolonged periods it is best to taper slowly, so that the body's own adrenal glands resume production of steroid.

When tapering the dose of steroids, one has to watch out for reappearance of the signs and symptoms of the disease and evidence of adrenal insufficiency or the ability for the adrenal glands to do their normal job. Symptoms include general fatigue or low blood pressure. The reduction of steroids and cortisol is associated with withdrawal and symptoms of aching muscles, bones, and joints.

During periods of extreme stress, the adrenal glands must produce large amounts of cortisol necessary to maintain normal physiological function. After prolonged oral doses of steroids, the glands are suppressed and do not produce large enough amounts in response to stress. During the perioperative period of surgery in those individuals, it is necessary to give extra intravenous doses of steroids for the stress and make up the difference of what the gland is not capable. Adrenal suppression continues as long as one year after discontinuing prolonged chronic oral steroid usage.

Steroids are given in divided doses throughout the day, then eventually twice a day, with the larger dose in the morning and the smaller dose in the evening, for example 5 mg each day in the A.M. and 2.5 mg each day in the P.M.

All chronic steroid users should carry identification describing their disease and steroid dose.

Anti-Inflammatory Effect

Because of their profound effect on inflammation, steroids are by far and away the most potent anti-inflammatory agents known to man. Since 1949, there have been few, if any, more important discoveries in the drug management of arthritis. The side effects associated with steroids have been a motivating force behind research to find better and safer drug therapies in the treatment of arthritis.

Other anti-inflammatories are generally referred to as nonsteroidal anti-inflammatories because they do not contain steroids. These drugs have a completely different profile of benefit versus risk. The number of NSAIDs has grown tremendously the last several years. NSAIDs can often be stopped if steroids are given concurrently. This avoids added risk.

There are many clinics just south of the Mexican border where American citizens seek out relief of their arthritis. Often the medications prescribed from these clinics include NSAIDs combined with steroids. Although there is initial relief for some patients, in the long run many return home to find out that the eventual side effects of steroids are worse than the disease.

Initiation of Steroids

Oral steroids may be started at any time during the course of arthritis or other forms of rheumatic illness. If the major "breadwinner" of a family develops severe progressive rheumatoid arthritis and can no longer bring home a paycheck to feed and care for the rest of the family, it is obviously time to start steroids. Steroids provide enough relief until other drug therapies with fewer side effects become effective. There is no evidence that steroids provide more than symptomatic relief in the treatment of rheumatoid arthritis.

Steroids bridge the gap and allow a breadwinner to continue to work. The decision to start oral steroid therapy is an important one!

Some patients are never able to taper and discontinue steroids. Long-term low-dose steroids are required to suppress the inflammation, regardless of alternative treatment programs. Low dose steroids are defined by less than or equal to 10 mg of prednisone or an equivalent steroid daily.

In other serious rheumatic disease states like vasculitis or SLE, high-dose steroid use is required to suppress the immunologic responses of the body that are part of the disease state. Although incompletely understood, once there is good suppression, steroids are safely tapered to lower levels. Steroids in this case disrupt the inflammatory cycle and allow a more normal state of health to return on less steroid. High-dose steroids are defined by more than 40 mg of prednisone or an equivalent steroid daily.

Because both response and side effects of steroids are dependent on dose size and the duration of treatment, it is crucial not to change doses without close monitoring by a physician and not to accept the attitude that more is better.

Every effort should be made to limit the use of steroids to the shortest course of time, and if maintenance treatment is necessary the lowest possible dosage that works.

Doses

The dose of steroid is important. Large doses are necessary to suppress serious life-threat-ening disease, yet smaller doses minimize side effects. Regardless of dose, steroids taken long enough will cause at least some side effects, especially thinning of the skin and bruising of the forearms. In postmenopausal women, it is important to try to keep the dose below 7.5 mg each day to minimize bone loss and osteoporosis. All patients on prolonged steroid doses for whatever reason, should have a baseline bone density done by DEXA methodology. Prophylactic addition of calcium and vitamin D supplements, along with an antiresorptive agent like an estrogen preparation, a bisphosphanate like alendronate (Fosamax) or risedronate (Actonel), raloxifene (Evista), or calcitonin (Miacalcin Nasal Spray) should be considered.

Several dosing schemes have been utilized to taper steroids, including decreasing the dose in an alternate day fashion. One day a larger dose is taken, the next day a smaller dose is taken in a continuous alternating regime. Every few weeks, one of the day's total doses is decreased while leaving the other day's dose alone. Eventually, steroids are given one day and off the next and so on.

Disease Modifying Antirheumatic Drugs

DMARDs or disease modifying antirheumatic drugs, remittive agents, or second-line drugs have the potential to reduce or prevent joint damage. While NSAIDs and steroids effectively alleviate symptoms, joint damage still occurs. All of these agents are used in several of the rheumatic illnesses; however, most of the following discussion pertains to RA. Some of these agents are used in combination.

Patients who have active persistent rheumatoid disease or who, early, during the course of their disease, have poor prognostic indicators are candidates for DMARDs. Poor prognostic indicators include those patients who despite adequate treatment with NSAIDs, have persistent fatigue and morning stiffness, those patients with persistent elevated markers of inflammation, as an elevated erythrocyte sedimentation rate (ESR) or C-reactive protein (CRP), and those patients with persistent swelling and signs of inflammation of the joints need early and aggressive treatment with DMARDs.

The decision to start a DMARD must be preceded by a discussion with the patient and close relatives or significant others about the risks versus benefits of the treatment and the expected outcome.

The best initial DMARD choice is not known, however, there are some advantages to each.

DISEASE MODIFYING ANTIRHEUMATIC DRUG THERAPY

- Sulfur medications (Azulfidine)
- Methotrexate (Rheumatrex)
- Gold therapy (Solganol, Aurolate)
- D-penicillamine (Depen, Cuprimine)
- Cyclosporine (Neoral)
- Leflunomide (Arava)
- Etanercept (Enbrel)
- Infliximab (Remicade)
- Prosorba Column
- Experimentals

Antimalarials

Because of the relative cost, safety, and convenience, antimalarials are often the initial selection for patients with mild disease of RA or SLE. At about four to six months, the effects of these drugs can usually be determined. The need for continuation of antimalarials or further drug therapies is then decided.

Antimalarials have been around a long time, since they were first used in the 1940s to treat malaria. Many years later, it was discovered that antimalarials were useful in the treatment of rheumatoid arthritis and systemic lupus erythematosus.

Antimalarials block ultraviolet light from damaging skin and have an anti-inflammatory effect. Interference with the immune response partly explains the beneficial effects. Unlike steroids and immunosuppressive agents, there is no adverse effect on blood counts, neither is there an increased risk for infection. Very little blood monitoring is necessary. Individuals who live in remote areas and have a difficult time going to the lab or doctor regularly, need not be seen frequently for the monitoring of this therapy.

In SLE, antimalarials are particularly effective in treating the skin rash, arthritis, or serositis. Serositis includes inflammation of the lining of the lung cavity or pleuritis, inflammation of the sack around the heart called pericarditis, or inflammation of the abdominal cavity. Antimalarials are steroid-sparing. Patients requiring steroids use less daily steroid doses than those individuals that do not take antimalarials at the same time. Antimalarials help many of the constitutional symptoms too, like fatigue or malaise. These compounds do not have a role in the treatment of more serious manifestations of SLE, especially central nervous system disease involvement of the brain and nerves or nephritis, which is kidney inflammation.

The two common oral preparations include hydroxychloroquine (Plaquenil) and chloroquine (Aralen). A third preparation quinacrine (Atabrine) is not associated with the side effects of the eye like hydroxychloroquine, but is associated with yellow pigmentation of the skin. Hydroxychloroquine is the only current antimalarial approved by the FDA and promoted specifically for RA. Chloroquine works more quickly, is more potent, but is not as safe as hydroxychloroquine. Quinacrine works quicker than hydroxychloroquine. Antimalarials cause some patients to experience headaches, muscle aches, and weakness. Stomach upset, loss of appetite, bloating, cramps, nausea and vomiting occur, but are infrequent and minor. Generally, antimalarial therapy is well tolerated.

The most important side effect of concern is possible damage to the back of the eye or retina. The retina can easily be seen during an eye exam by the eye specialist. The macula of the eye can be damaged by antimalarials. The macular changes as a consequence of antimalarial drug therapy is dose-related on a daily basis and rarely, if ever, occurs if hydroxychloroquine is given at a maximum of 400 mg a day or less. If the dose is kept below this level, effects on the eye are most unusual. If treated early, this side effect on the retina reverses without loss of vision. Treatment of the eye problem requires early discontinuation of the antimalarial.

As with most medicines, more antimalarial therapy is not necessarily better. Examination of the retina before treatment and every six months is suggested. Routine eye exams by an ophthalmologist including color vision and visual fields detect early or mild changes that are more apt to be reversible.

The beneficial effects of antimalarials in both RA and SLE take several weeks to work. Antimalarials are slow-acting drugs. Side effects have been reported to occur weeks after the medicine is discontinued. It is important to stop this medicine several months before pregnancy, since it has an ill effect on a fetus or newborn baby, and can result in deafness. Generally, antimalarials are well tolerated. Most patients starting the medicine will continue. Only a small percentage ever experience any difficulty with antimalarials.

Plaquenil is the most commonly prescribed antimalarial. Tablets of 200 mg each are given twice a day after a normal eye exam. Unless not tolerated, the dose is kept at this amount for several months. After the patient is stabilized and doing better, Plaquenil can be stopped altogether, if not needed, or tapered slowly over many weeks. Switching from seven days a week to five days a week, and later before stopping altogether, three days a week, is one method of discontinuing the medicine. Dosing is always twice a day and never more. Variations of this dose schedule are utilized. Just as the effects of antimalarials take weeks to occur, once these drugs are stopped the effects are not lost for weeks. Therefore, missing a dose or two will have no immediate effect on the disease course, unless missed often. Antimalarials are regarded as safe to use in the treatment of rheumatoid arthritis or SLE.

Sulfur Medications

Sulfasalazine (Azulfidine or Azulfidine EN) is a sulfa drug that for many years has been used in the treatment of inflammatory conditions of the bowel. Azulfidine has been available since the late 1940s. It seems to have both an anti-inflammatory effect like aspirin compounds and an antibiotic effect in the treatment of gastrointestinal disorders. This compound should not be taken by those people allergic to sulfa medications. Azulfidine is given early in RA or in combination with other remittive agents. Periodic blood monitoring is required for those individuals

on these drugs. Although there are a number of serious side effects, they are for the most part, not serious, and are readily reversible. Common side effects include headache, nausea, diarrhea, rash, and on occasion low blood counts. Men experience a low sperm count that appears to be reversible upon discontinuation of the medicine. The tendency has been to use sulfasalazine in refractory cases, but in these situations it works less well, than other remittive drugs. It is best to use it early in cases of RA that respond inadequately to NSAIDs. It is used in conjunction with both NSAIDs, steroids, and some remittive agents. This drug demonstrates clinical response after a relatively short treatment period of about one to three months. Periodic blood tests are necessary to monitor for side effects.

The tablets are each 500 mg and given in divided doses twice, three, or even four times a day. A maximum total daily dose is about 3,000 mg daily. Azulfidine EN-Tabs are enteric coated to reduce stomach absorption and minimize gastrointestinal irritation. This is intended to reduce the possibility of stomach upset, such as nausea and vomiting.

Methotrexate

Rheumatologists select methotrexate (Rheumatrex) as the initial DMARD most of the time, especially for patients with severe disease and who need a quick response. Methotrexate (MTX) appears to have the most predictable benefit and patients stay on it longer than any other DMARD. The fact that MTX can induce cancers like lymphoma in a small number of RA patients remains a concern not well proven, nevertheless, it requires a continued awareness of its potential on rare occasions.

Many would agree that one of the most meaningful advances in the treatment of RA over the past decade or more has been the acceptance and increasingly widespread use of methotrexate. Although first developed to treat certain cancers, in 1988 MTX was approved by the FDA for the treatment of RA. Clinical rheumatologists have widely accepted the use of MTX in the treatment of RA ever since. MTX is the most commonly used second-line agent for the treatment of RA. MTX's original design was to interfere with folate and act as a chemotherapeutic agent in the treatment of cancer. Clearly, MTX is as effective in patients as other anti-rheumatic drugs including Plaquenil, gold, and penicillamine. Despite well-known adverse experiences, the drug is tolerated by most patients. Patients usually improve rapidly in a few weeks, plateau at about six months, and then are maintained.

Careful attention must be directed toward adjusting dose levels of the therapy. Frequent individualized dosage manipulations are necessary to allow the drug to be contin-ued safely. It is likely that the initial dose of MTX will have to be changed because of a side effect that may or may not be noticed by the patient. Toxicity appears to be more common in the higher dose range. A 7.5 mg weekly dose represents an appropriate initial starting level for most patients. The average dose is usually 15 mg weekly, but higher doses are used.

Methotrexate is given weekly rather than daily; the weekly dose is taken either singularly or in divided doses.

For MTX to be assigned its proper role in the treatment of RA, its long-term safety must be demonstrated in the face of its enthusiasm.

Investigations, especially with patients who have psoriasis, suggest an incidence of fibrosis and cirrhosis or scarring of the liver. Blood monitoring of liver function on a routine chemistry panel is an indirect look at the liver as compared to a liver biopsy. Current recommendations for liver biopsy are for those individuals who develop liver function blood abnormalities that persist during treatment with or after the discontinuation of the drug. A liver biopsy is usually not recommended before therapy with MTX. The chemical analysis of liver function through blood tests may or may not be able to detect inflammation of the liver before important abnormalities occur.

Those patients already at an increased risk for liver disease, including alcoholics with cirrhosis, should not take MTX.

Alcohol consumption is not absolutely forbidden, but should be minimized or avoided if possible. If any abnormalities of liver function occur with MTX treatment, alcohol should be stopped immediately and the blood analysis done again. Regular blood monitoring is mandatory. Individuals with hepatitis C should probably avoid MTX.

Other important reported side effects of MTX include minimal hair loss, a low blood count, nausea, and inflammation of the lining of the mouth. Potentially dangerous lung inflammation induced by MTX is fortunately unusual, but is very serious. Some of the adverse effects are life threatening, but tend to be less frequent at lower doses or require temporary discontinuance of therapy. The concurrent use of folate or folic acid daily doesn't seem to interfere with the beneficial effects of the drug and diminishes some of the side effects, since folate is depleted while taking MTX. Folic acid 1 mg a day is readily available by prescription, or smaller amounts in inexpensive once-a-day multivitamins.

An interesting problem associated with MTX therapy is an exacerbation or induction of rheumatoid nodules in a small number of patients with RA; even when substantial anti-inflammatory effects are achieved from the drug. This is more common if there are preexisting nodules. The reason for nodulosis is poorly understood and in some cases necessitates the discontinuation of MTX, surgery, or the addition of other drugs. Antimalarials or sulfasalazine help reduce the nodulosis.

Aspirin and other NSAIDs are used with MTX; however, the potential for interaction should be watched. Steroids are continued and then gradually reduced once a response to MTX is obtained. Concomitant use of other DMARDs has been studied. In some refractory patients not responding to MTX therapy, combination DMARDs are helpful. Cyclosporine and anti-TNF drug therapy are beneficial in combination with MTX.

MTX is given as a single oral dose once weekly or in divided doses at twelve-hour intervals for a maximum of three doses weekly. It is also be given by self-injection once a week.

The importance of taking doses on a weekly basis should be emphasized.

The dosage of MTX is reduced to the least possible amount of drug once response is achieved. Improvement begins within three to six weeks in contrast to other DMARDs that take twelve to sixteen weeks to show response. Injectable doses of MTX are self-administered at home with a small needle subcutaneously and have several advantages. Injectable MTX is currently less expensive than oral tablets. Liver toxicity is less with injectable MTX than oral tablets. Injectable MTX initially bypasses the liver until after it goes to the tissues. The liver actually sees lower concentrations of drug than when taken orally. The initial bypass of the liver can eventually allow higher doses of MTX by injection if necessary to control the arthritis. Most injectable dose levels used are similar to the oral doses.

Methotrexate should not be taken by people with serious kidney or liver disease, who drink alcohol, or who have AIDS. Women of childbearing potential must practice contraception and it should never be taken during pregnancy.

MTX is not associated with the acute sickness that occurs with therapy given to cancer patients. Immunosuppression does put one at risk for an increased incidence of infection and susceptibility to unusual infections that would not otherwise be a problem in a healthy individual with a normal immune system. The potential to induce malignancy after prolonged periods of therapy requires a constant vigilance. The problems of infection or increased potential for cancer are both related to the suppression of the immune system, which benefits the disease. Because of the chance of serious adverse effects, these drugs must be kept out of the reach of small children and not given to women of childbearing potential. MTX may cause birth defects if taken at the time of conception or during pregnancy. MTX should be avoided during concurrent infections or the flu.

Women of childbearing potential must use birth control and not become pregnant while taking MTX.

MTX has no effect on fertility in women. MTX has been given to women with ectopic pregnancy to induce abortion. Men may experience lower sperm counts temporarily, until MTX is discontinued.

Another immunosuppressive drug is azathioprine or Imuran. Imuran is used less frequently than MTX. This drug is well tolerated, but initially requires frequent and close monitoring of the blood counts because of suppression of the number of white cells. Later, as the dose is stabilized, the cell counts are done less often. The correct dose needed to suppress the disease is often judged by at least some suppression of the white cell count.

Gold Therapy

Intramuscular gold injections have been utilized for many years. Weekly injections for several months are required before beginning less frequent injections and eventual monthly maintenance therapy. Monitoring of blood and urine is required before each and every injection. Oral gold preparations like auranofin (Ridaura) do not appear to be effective and are rarely used. There are currently two available gold preparations given by intramuscular injection. These include an oil-based gold, aurothioglucose (Solganol), which is absorbed slowly from the muscle, and another faster absorbed preparation, gold sodium thiomalate (Aurolate). The fast absorption of a gold injection may be associated with lightheadedness or dizziness as result of a drop in the blood pressure. This effect occurs as a consequence of the dilatation of blood vessels similar to taking nitroglycerin and is called a nitritoid reaction. This doesn't seem to occur with the slower absorbing preparation. For that reason, aurothioglucose may be safer in older individuals who cannot afford a drop in blood pressure.

The very first gold injection should be a small test dose.

Gold injections are given in the buttocks. Seldom do patients complain about the shot, but rather the required blood monitoring and frequent doctor visits at the initiation of therapy. Gold injections are cumbersome because of the initial frequency, monitoring, and potential side effects. Unfortunately, there is no test available to determine who will respond or develop side effects.

All of the side effects of gold therapy are reversible if the patient is supported and waits long enough. Even so, many are very serious and life-threatening and require that the medication be stopped immediately and never restarted. Dry, scaly and itchy rashes are common and usually a nuisance. Rashes improve with lower doses of gold, delaying the frequency of injection, or applying topical steroid creams. Itching is helped by antihistamines. Extreme skin reactions and rash occur infrequently. Decreases in the blood count occur commonly and are monitored closely before each injection of gold. Diminished platelet counts result in excessive bruising. A low white cell count increases the chance for infection and should be avoided. An irritation of the kidney results in leakage of protein into the urine and can be extreme. Protein is discovered early by monitoring with a urinary dipstick and usually reverses without harm to kidney function.

D-Penicillamine

D-penicillamine (Cuprimine, Depen) is also effective. It is not utilized as much now because of the popularity of other DMARDs. Dosing is a little inconvenient, and requires a "go low and go slow" regime, that is, changes in doses are made infrequently. More individuals will quit penicillamine because of side effects than gold injections, but just as many will respond too. Penicillamine has most of the same side effects as gold therapy plus others, including a lupus-like syndrome. Loss of taste may occur. Penicillamine can be given to penicillin allergic individuals.

It takes months for penicillamine to take effect. It is important to continue taking the medicine for a period of time to determine effectiveness. Stopping and starting medicine increases the chance for ill effects from the drug. Medication as 250 mg tablets or capsules is taken on an empty stomach two hours before or after meals. The medication is taken once a day or in divided doses as the total dose each day is increased. Few patients get better on 250 mg per day. The maximum daily dose is 1500 mg per day.

Cyclosporine

Cyclosporine (Sandimmune, Neoral) is an immunomodulating agent approved for the treatment of RA. This drug has made organ transplantation possible. It is a drug that has significant effects on the immune system. Its long-term efficacy and toxicity in RA remains unclear. Disadvantages include costs relative to other second-line agents and potential kidney dysfunction and toxicity. During organ transplantation of heart, liver, or kidney the immunologic benefits of cyclosporine justify its indefinite use, even if some kidney dysfunction occurs. In contrast to organ transplantation the dose used for the treatment of autoimmune disease is lower. However, some patients with RA require

prolonged treatment and kidney toxicity is of concern. Cyclosporine should not be given to individuals with any preexisting kidney disease or hypertension. The kidney function of patients with rheumatic diseases taking cyclosporine must be monitored, since both the disease and drug therapy impact kidney function. The evaluation of kidney function includes the monitoring of blood pressure, blood, and urine tests. If blood tests determine kidney function worsens by thirty percent compared to tests done at the initiation of therapy, the dose must be reduced. Kidney toxicity is manageable, but not negligible. NSAIDs work in concert with regards to kidney toxicity and depress kidney function. Withdrawal of NSAIDs is not always feasible.

Besides the adverse effects on the kidney, other side effects include extra facial hair growth, acne, diarrhea, nausea and vomiting, and swelling of the gums around the teeth.

Whether DMARDs should be given sequentially or additively for patients remains controversial, however the trend is to use these drugs in combination now more than years past. In many patients with severe RA who partially respond to MTX, combination therapy with cyclosporine and MTX results in clinically important improvement compared with MTX alone.

The rationale for the use of cyclosporine depends on the role of T-cell function and cellular immunity as compared to B-cell function and humeral immunity. Together cellular and humeral immunity make up the immune response. In RA, there is abundant evidence for the role of T-cells in the inflammatory process; on the other hand, in systemic lupus erythematosus humeral immunity is more important than cellular immunity. Therefore, there is less rationale for the use of cyclosporine in SLE.

Remission does not appear to be seen in response to this drug therapy. Cyclosporine does appear to reduce inflammation, pain, and improve mobility. In kidney transplant patients, cyclosporine is associated with an increased frequency of cancer. It generally takes between four and eight weeks for symptomatic relief.

Cyclosporine is given in liquid form or more palatable soft gelatin capsules. The capsules come in 25-mg or 100-mg sizes. The dose is split and given twice a day. The dose is dependent upon weight. For the average individual low doses are 150–200 mg/day. At low doses, side effects are mostly reversible. Grapefruit and grapefruit juice should be avoided within an hour of the medication, since it can alter the absorption of the medication.

Leflunomide

Leflunomide (Arava) was the first in a number of new rheumatoid arthritis medicines to hit the market. Leflunomide is not a cure. The drug works by blocking the overproduction of immune cells that are responsible for the inflammation caused by arthritis. Early studies have shown just about as much improvement as methotrexate in comparison to placebo. Side effects include diarrhea, rash, hair loss, and liver toxicity. Patients need regular blood monitoring, especially the liver. Any toxicity typically occurs soon after patients begin taking the drug.

For women, leflunomide has special warnings. Women must not get pregnant while leflunomide is still in their body. Women taking leflunomide must use effective birth control while taking the medicine, since animal studies suggest the drug can cause numerous birth defects. Unlike most drugs that rapidly clear out of the body after the last dose is taken, leflunomide can linger for months. Women who wish to become pregnant can take an anticholesterol drug called cholestyramine to help flush leflunomide out of their bloodstream before conception. To minimize any risk for birth defects, men wishing to father a child should also consider discontinuing the use of leflunomide and take cholestyramine. The manufacturers have devised an elimination procedure if leflunomide must be stopped. A full eleven-day course of cholestyramine medication is followed by two separate laboratory blood tests at least fourteen days apart to insure a very low drug level in your body. If the drug levels are too high, a repeated drug elimination procedure is necessary. After the drug elimination procedure, the risk of having a baby with birth defects is very low and should be no higher than the risk in the general population. Without the elimination procedure, it could take up to two years to reach a very low level of leflunomide in the blood.

Because blood levels increase slowly, the first three days of leflunomide is given as a 100-mg tablet daily then 20 mg a day, thereafter. If side effects are suspected, the dose can be reduced to 10 mg per day. Leflunomide does not require dose increases, although lower doses are used if tolerability is a problem. The drug is taken without regard to meals or the concomitant use of NSAIDs or steroids.

A positive effect is evident by one month and stabilized by three to six months, then continues throughout treatment. Studies of x-rays have suggested a slowing of disease progression.

Etanercept

Etanercept (Enbrel) is a protein and is produced by recombinant DNA technology in a hamster. Etanercept binds specifically to tumor necrosis factor (TNF) and blocks its action. TNF is a natural occurring chemical in the body that promotes the inflammatory and immune responses. TNF plays an especially important role in the inflammatory processes of rheumatoid arthritis and the resulting joint damage. Elevated levels of TNF are found in the joint fluid of RA patients. Etanercept is given as a small injection twice a week at home by the patient. The first injections are performed under the supervision of a health care provider. The ability to give a safe subcutaneous injection must be assessed. The medicine comes as a powder in a vial. Sterile water is added to the powder and the medicine dissolves. Responses appear within two weeks after initiation of therapy and nearly always by three months. After discontinuation of medicine symptoms of arthritis return within a month. Currently, etanercept is recommended for those RA patients with symptoms of moderate-to-severe disease who have had an inadequate response to one or more disease-modifying antirheumatic drugs. Etanercept can be used in conjunction with more recognized therapies like methotrexate. Allergic reactions to etanercept have been rare, although itching or rash at the injection site can occur. The long-term effects of anti-TNF medications are not known, especially with the body's defense mechanisms against infection or malignancies. Patients who develop a new infection while undergoing treatment with etanercept should be monitored closely. Treatment should be discontinued in patients with serious infections. Other side effects occur infrequently, but include headache, nasal congestion, dizziness, sore throat, cough, weakness, abdominal pain, rash, lung problems, shortness of breath, or inflammation of the sinuses. Early reports have demonstrated possible exacerbations in multiple sclerosis patients.

Infliximab

A second anti-tumor necrosis factor is infliximab (Remicade). Infliximab also works by neutralizing the biological activity of tumor necrosis factor. Infliximab works quickly and a patient with RA can feel substantially better within two weeks of the first therapy. In a yearlong study of continued treatment with infliximab, relief continued and as was long lasting.

The medicine is diluted in fluid and given as an intravenous infusion. This simple procedure is routinely performed in doctors' offices and other medical facilities. After the initial dose is repeated at two weeks and six weeks, treatment is given once every eight weeks or six times a year. It is effective treatment and provides relief for the entire eight weeks between treatments. The treatment is well tolerated. The most common side effects include upper respiratory infections, headache, nausea, coughing, and diarrhea. Very few people stop the treatment because of side effects.

Infliximab is a monoclonal antibody. This antibody was developed to accurately and specifically target tumor necrosis factor or TNF. Medical studies have shown that infliximab effectively relieves the signs and symptoms of RA with methotrexate.

The solution of infliximab is given intravenously as an infusion slowly over about two hours. The dose is carefully calculated based on the weight of the patient. During the infusion the vital signs including pulse, blood pressure, and temperature are monitored. During the period of the infusion, patients can relax, read a book, listen to music, or even watch TV. Some people notice mild reactions like itching or a stinging feeling, and rarely chills, difficulty breathing, or low blood pressure. When reactions occur, they resolve if the treatment is stopped or temporarily slowed down. Subsequent infusion reactions necessitate premedicating with acetaminophen or antihistamines. If no premedications are given, the patient can resume a normal schedule following the infusion.

All TNF-blocking agents and concomitant immunosuppressive therapy alter the immune response, including the response to infection. Those individuals with chronic infections or a history of recurring infection should probably avoid anti-TNF treatment. There is a concern about inducing cancers. Although clinically cancer has not been a problem, close monitoring occurs.

Prosorba Column

This medical device received approval by the FDA for the treatment of RA in those individuals for whom other treatments have provided little help. The device is the size of a soup can and filters harmful immune complexes from the bloodstream. The procedure is done weekly for twelve weeks. Each session lasts about two hours per treatment. Almost one-half of the treated patients in clinical studies got improvement that lasted twenty to seventy-five weeks. The projected cost and time commitment for this procedure make it an undesirable option for some people. The procedure is approved for people with moderate-to-severe RA who have not experienced significant relief from methotrexate or at least two other DMARDs.

Experimentals or Biologicals

Research for new drugs in the treatment of RA and other rheumatic illnesses is keen. New drugs show promise in blocking the biological processes that perpetuate the joint inflammation and destruction of joints. Several drugs that can block cytokines or mediators of inflammation like IL-1 are currently under investigation. In the normal immune system these cytokines are thought to regulate pro-inflammatory activity and contribute to the arthritis and inflammatory state.

Goals of Treatment

The goal of treatment with DMARDs is to begin early and prevent joint damage. The diagnosis of RA must be certain. On occasion this is difficult, and the natural course of the disease must be observed. Few other conditions than RA are appropriate to treat with remittive agents, although their usefulness is expanding in other rheumatic conditions.

All DMARDs are slow in acting. There is no blood test to determine who will respond or who will have a reaction. Efficacy is determined on an individualized basis and each and every patient must be monitored carefully for side effects. Each DMARD is unique. The choice of DMARD depends on the need for convenience, the requirements for monitoring, the cost of medications, the time until expected benefit, the frequency of side effects, other medications or complicating medical problems, previous experience of the patient and physician, and finally the ability to comply.

Nonsteroidal Anti-Inflammatory Drugs

NSAIDs are the most commonly prescribed class of drugs. They are used in all forms of arthritis. More than 70 million prescriptions for NSAIDs are written annually in the United States. Seventeen million Americans take NSAIDs on a regular basis. Over ten percent of the population older than sixty-five years of age use NSAIDs.

"NSAIDs are one of the safest and most effective classes of medications ever developed for arthritis. Despite their remarkable safety however, their use has been plagued by gastrointestinal side effects. Side effects range from mild pain, gastric ulcers, to life-threatening internal bleeding. In the future, COX-2 selective inhibitors may offer more safety for patients that require medications for arthritis pain control."

William R. Brugge, M.D.
Harvard Medical School
Massachusetts General Hospital
Boston, Massachusetts

Examples of available NSAIDs include: ibuprofen (Motrin, Advil, Nuprin, Medipren), naproxen (Naprosyn, Aleve, Naprelan), sulindac (Clinoril), diclofenac (Voltaren, Voltaren XR), piroxicam (Feldene), ketoprofen (Orudis, Oruvail), diflunical (Dolobid), nabumetone (Relafen), etodolac (Lodine, Lodine XL), oxaprozim (Daypro), indomethacin (Indocin, Indocin SR), and others. In low doses, many of these medications are available at the drugstore over the counter.

TYPES OF NONSTEROIDAL ANTI-INFLAMMATORIES

- Traditional anti-inflammatories by prescription
- Traditional anti-inflammatories over the counter
- COX 2 selective agents
- Aspirin or aspirin-like medications

NSAID Gastropathy

The major concern of NSAIDs for the treatment of arthritis patients is the incidence of stomach problems. Inflammation of the lining of the stomach wall caused by these medications creates ulceration or erosions that results in internal bleeding. The term NSAID gastropathy has been adopted and it is discovered by upper gastrointestinal endoscopy. Upper GI endoscopy is the passage of a scope through the mouth and into the esophagus, stomach, and the duodenum and allows direct visualization and biopsy of the stomach wall if necessary. Although, only a small percentage of NSAID users ever develop serious complications of ulcer disease, it is still estimated that more than 10,000 deaths occur annually secondary to these drugs. The development of a safer NSAID has become increasingly more important since we have become aware of these complications.

Mechanism of Action

NSAIDs are regarded by many as the foundation of drug treatment for inflammatory arthritis. A large number of NSAIDs are approved by the Food and Drug Administration (FDA) for use in the United States. Most NSAIDs inhibit the formation of a group of substances called prostaglandins, which are mediators of inflammation. Preventing the formation of prostaglandins lessens the pain and inflammation of arthritis. Although most of these medications work in the same fashion, there are differences between them, and some are better tolerated than others.

Side Effects

The benefits and side effects vary from patient to patient. Side effects noticed by one individual may not be noticed by someone else taking the same drug for the same reason. Likewise, benefits experienced by one person may not be experienced by another. Sometimes, the drug will stop working, even though it did well for a while. Manufacturers of drugs have pursued different indications for their NSAIDs with the FDA to make their products unique. While some differences in the chemistry among NSAIDs do exist, there is limited information on the practical consequences of such differences.

NSAIDs may have less toxicity than salicylates, or aspirin-like medications. However, they are not without problems, particularly in elderly patients. Adverse effects include stomach ulcers, the inability of the kidney to function normally, congestive heart failure from fluid retention, bleeding and the aggravation of hypertension. Central nervous system toxicity occurs resulting in poor memory, fatigue, reduced concentration, depression, and headache. NSAID therapy should be avoided in patients with a history of gastrointestinal or kidney disease and monitored more carefully in the elderly.

Less common side effects include skin rashes, abnormal liver function tests, asthma and severe headache and neck stiffness that resembles meningitis. The majority of NSAID-related side effects are reversible once the drug is stopped. During continued use, regular blood counts, as well as liver and kidney function should be monitored every three or four months.

In most instances, it is not a good idea to combine different NSAIDs. Even so, on occasion salicylates are combined. Together however, this increases the chance of side effects. Salicylates are nonsteroidal anti-inflammatories that are really part of the aspirin family. Nonacetylated salicylates (Disalcid or Trilisate) minimize some of the side effects of acetylated salicylates like aspirin. Nonacetylated salicylates have no effect on platelets, whereas aspirin decreases the stickiness of platelets and thins the blood. Platelets are a component of the blood that plug up the holes in the circulation when we bleed. Thinning of the blood from NSAIDs only occurs while actually taking the medication, and doesn't last as long as the same effects of aspirin. One aspirin thins the blood for several weeks. Even small doses of aspirin affect bleeding times. For that reason, heart patients often take one 81-mg or baby aspirin a day. Most nonacetylated salicylates are taken less often than aspirin tablets. The usual full anti-inflammatory dose of aspirin is three tablets four times a day with food. Larger doses usually result in ringing in the ears called tinnitus, or upset stomach like heartburn or dyspepsia. Some individuals tolerate even higher doses of daily aspirin.

An advantage of aspirin therapy is the ability to measure therapeutic blood levels.

Most benefits of NSAIDs are on the basis of the inhibition of hormones within the body called prostaglandins, so are the side effects. Unfortunately, these medications cannot sort out or differentiate "good" from "bad" prostaglandins. Therefore, both are inhibited; upsetting the normal balance of protective mechanisms of the body. Prostaglandins protect the stomach wall from injury as a result of normal acid production. The ability of prostaglandins in the stomach wall to protect from ulceration is eliminated after the use of NSAIDs.

Stomach Ulcers

Several medications help heal or prevent stomach ulcers and may be taken concurrently with anti-inflammatories, including cimetidine (Tagamet), ranitidine (Zantac), sulcrafate (Carafate), omeprazole (Prilosec), and lansoprazole (Prevacid). Except for sulcrafate, all of these medications stop or decrease the production of stomach acid, some more than others. These medications in small doses have become available over the counter. Several medications help heal or prevent stomach ulcers and may be taken concurrently with anti-inflammatories. Misoprostol (Cytotec) has the ability to put synthetic protective prostaglandins back into the stomach wall and defend the stomach from its own acid production. Acid production is not altered. Cytotec causes diarrhea, uterine cramping, and must be avoided in women of childbearing potential because of its effects on the uterus. The concurrent use of misoprostol with NSAIDs definitely decreases the chance of developing stomach ulcers. Drugs like cimetidine (Tagamet) or rantidine (Zantac) decrease the production of stomach acid. Omeprazole (Prilosec) and similar drugs totally block the acid secretion altogether. Sulcrafate helps heal ulcers. Additional risk factors for ulcer disease or its complications include smoking, alcohol consumption, and the concurrent use of steroids and other medications, including blood thinners like coumadin. There is concern that the medicines that prevent acid formation may cover up symptoms and put the patient at an increased risk for GI bleeding. Cytotec would be an exception, since it replaces the protective prostaglandins in the stomach wall and does not inhibit acid production. An individual can develop damage to the stomach lining without being aware of it. There may be no history or nausea, vomiting, or diarrhea. Even gastrointestinal bleeding occurs frequently without any early symptoms.

Various delivery modes have been attempted to get around GI distress with the anti-inflammatories, including enteric coatings or time-released preparations. Ecotrin is an enteric-coated aspirin. Enteric coatings prevent breakdown of NSAIDs in the stomach, and allow release of the medication farther down the GI tract. The benefits of enteric coatings are minimal, since the more important effect of the NSAIDs is its effects through the bloodstream and the depletion of the stomach prostaglandins. Food provides similar and minimal benefit.

Symptomatic Therapy

NSAIDs are often utilized in the treatment of musculoskeletal pain and inflammation and are well tolerated. They are used in conjunction with other medications in the treatment of more serious rheumatic illnesses, but do not have the ability to suppress the immune system (immunosuppressive), and therefore, are symptomatic treatments only.

Anti-inflammatories do not change the course of arthritis. They are symptomatic treatment only.

NSAIDs in low doses are used for their analgesic properties, that is their ability to ease pain and not their anti-inflammatory effects. In low doses NSAIDs are available over the counter at the pharmacy without the need for a prescription.

Aspirin

There are several different preparations of aspirin. Regular aspirin is usually a tablet of 5 grains or 325 milligrams. It is inexpensive. Dressed-up aspirin, "extra-strength" or "arthritis strength" can become more expensive. Buffered aspirin—aspirin surrounded with antacid—may be more expensive. Enteric-coated aspirin is encased in a shell that passes intact through the stomach to dissolve in the intestine. This is meant to protect the stomach. Sustained-release aspirin releases aspirin over several hours rather than the whole dose at once. Full anti-inflammatory doses of aspirin are usually twelve or more tablets of regular aspirin a day. Some individuals can handle even larger doses because of their metabolism. Most individuals experience ringing in the ears—tinnitus—when the aspirin in their blood approaches toxic levels. Unfortunately, in some elderly individuals, they cannot hear the ringing. If ringing occurs, the dose can be diminished by a ½ aspirin a day periodically, and once the ringing resolves that individual is close to a therapeutic level, but below the toxic level. The range between the toxic and therapeutic levels is very close and narrow, but blood levels can be measured if necessary.

Not surprisingly, aspirin has long been used by people with arthritis. Although it has had a bad rap in recent times, it may be one of the safest medicines, considering that Americans alone take millions of tablets a day.

Aspirin, like NSAIDs, block the production of prostaglandins, hormone-like substances that play a major role in the production of pain, inflammation, and fever. The full effects of aspirin take several days until a therapeutic level in the blood is achieved. In addition, aspirin has analgesic effects and lowers temperature effectively.

Side Effects

Aspirin can cause problems. Aspirin irritates the stomach lining and causes heartburn, indigestion, nausea, vomiting, and even bleeding, just like NSAIDs. Nonacetylated aspirin causes fewer stomach problems than plain aspirin. Allergic reactions occur rarely, but occur more commonly in those individuals with asthma and nasal polyps.

Aspirin interferes with clotting of the blood; its effects can last several weeks and cause bleeding in susceptible people. It should never be used by people with a history of ulcers of the stomach, since internal bleeding could be catastrophic. Yet, this same problem makes aspirin useful for those individuals threatened by stroke or heart attack. One daily aspirin tablet is rarely associated with problems, but is highly effective in thinning the blood. It is taken for prophylaxis against blood clots. The advantages far outweigh the risks. Those individuals who need to keep their blood thinned are less susceptible to clotting. For these same reasons, aspirin should be avoided prior to surgery, since it can increase the risk of unnecessary bleeding.

Aspirin is no do-it-yourself matter.

A qualified physician should supervise those individuals taking aspirin on a regular basis in large doses. It is important to read the labels of over-the-counter medications that contain aspirin. While aspirin is a wonder drug with a long and interesting history, it can be harmful and should be taken as part of a treatment program of arthritis prescribed by a physician. Alcohol should be avoided while taking aspirin, since alcohol can also irritate the stomach.

COX-2 Agents

One class of NSAIDs appears to have fewer side effects. These medications are more selective in the inhibition of enzymes active in the formation of mediators of inflammation, and are called COX-2 selective inhibitors. They are able to sort out the inhibition of "good" and "bad" prostaglandins. Inhibiting the "bad" prostaglandins benefits arthritis, while preserving the "good" prostaglandins. This maintains important protective mechanisms to the body and minimizes side effects, especially stomach ulcers. Celecoxib (Celebrex) and rofecoxib (Vioxx) are the first of several of these drugs released. Meloxicam (Mobic) has some COX-2 selectivity.

Cytotoxics

Cytotoxic drugs or immunosuppressive agents have been mentioned elsewhere. Their importance and significance deserve further mention, especially in the treatment of systemic lupus erythematosus (SLE) or other autoimmune disease. These medicines are very potent and help reduce disease activity in major organs like the kidney (nephritis). Immunosuppressive agents can be used either in addition to, or instead of steroids. They can be steroid-sparing, helping avoid the many side effects of steroid therapy. Although many of these drugs may have serious side effects, close monitoring avoids most trouble. These drugs can have significant benefits and can prolong life.

Mechanism of Action
Rapidly dividing cells in the body are most susceptible to the effects of chemotherapeutic drugs. Azathi-

COMMON IMMUNOSUPPRESSIVE AGENTS IN THE TREATMENT OF RHEUMATOID ARTHRITIS
• Azathioprine (Imuran)
• Cyclophosphamide (Cytoxan)
• Others

oprine (Imuran) and cyclophosphamide (Cytoxan) are utilized in autoimmune diseases. Other cytotoxic drugs include chlorambucil (Leukeran), nitrogen mustard (Mustargen), and methotrexate (Rheumatrex). Cytotoxic drugs work by targeting and damaging cells that grow at a rapid rate, primarily malignant cells, but also antibody-producing cells of the immune system, blood cells, hair cells, and reproductive cells like the ovaries and testes. In autoimmune diseases, these drugs work by suppressing the hyperactive cells of the immune system that are overworking.

Side Effects

The immune system may also be suppressed too much. This results in reductions of the cellular components of the blood stream including the red cells called anemia, white cells called leukopenia, or platelets called thrombocytopenia. Anemia may add to fatigue. Leukopenia increases the risk for infection and decreases ability to fight infections. Thrombocytopenia results in excess bleeding, since platelets are sticky and plug up holes in the bloodstream. Oversuppression of hair cells results in scalp baldness and loss of hair on other parts of the body too. The cytotoxic effects of the reproductive cells can result in difficulty conceiving or even sterility.

Blood cell counts monitor the effects of Imuran and should be taken regularly; more often at the initiation of therapy or change of dosing; less often—once a month—when a stable dose is reached. Suppression to some degree of the total white count is a good measure of the best dose. In most cases, Imuran is well tolerated. Experience with kidney-transplant patients suggests there might be a slight increased risk for new cancer in those patients taking higher doses for prolonged periods of time.

Cytoxan is more potent, and has the potential for greater side effects. The increased risk for cancer is more apparent and real in comparison to Imuran. These cancers may include leukemia, bladder cancer, and other tumors. Inflammation of the bladder (cystitis) may result in bleeding into the urine from the bladder. Large amounts of oral fluid intake during the treatment are important. Like Imuran, there may be an increased risk for infection, and sometimes unusual infections including shingles, a very painful blistering condition. Hair loss occurs with Cytoxan and temporary or permanent sterility may occur. Cytoxan can be given orally or intravenously.

Doses

Occasionally, large intravenous boluses of Cytoxan are given monthly several times in a row. This therapy is well tolerated and especially important in SLE patients with nephritis. Oral doses of either Imuran or Cytoxan on a daily basis requires periodic monitoring of the blood cell counts. A typical daily oral dose of Imuran or Cytoxan is similar and is usually about 100–200 milligrams (mg). Cytoxan is best taken in the morning with fluids during the day, and should never be taken with Imuran at the same time. Imuran is not given intravenously.

Immunosuppressive agents should not be used indefinitely, if possible. They must always be monitored closely. Written prescriptions should never be written without a time limit; for example, one month at a time. Although these drugs are the standard of practice in many autoimmune and rheumatic illnesses, an informed consent should be given by the prescribing physician. An informed consent includes a thorough discussion of the risks and benefits of such medicine.

CHAPTER 27

Biologicals

Biologicals include medications that neutralize a protein in the circulation important in the formation of inflammation. The effects tend to be quick and profound.

APPROVED BIOLOGICAL AGENTS
• Etanercept (Enbrel)
• Infliximab (Remicade)

Etanercept

Etanercept (Enbrel) is a genetically engineered protein produced by recombinant DNA technology in a hamster. Etanercept binds specifically to tumor necrosis factor (TNF) and blocks its action. TNF is a naturally occurring chemical in the body that promotes the inflammatory and immune responses. TNF plays an important role in the inflammatory processes of rheumatoid arthritis and the resulting joint damage. Elevated levels of TNF are found in the joint fluid of RA patients. Etanercept is given as a small subcutaneous injection twice a week at home by the patient. The first injections are performed under the supervision of a health-care provider. The ability to give a safe subcutaneous injection must be assessed. The medicine comes as a powder in a vial. Sterile water is added to the powder and the medicine dissolves. Responses appear within two weeks after initiation of therapy and nearly always by three months. After discontinuation of medicine, symptoms of arthritis return within a month. Etanercept is recommended for those RA patients with symptoms of moderate-to-severe disease who have had an inadequate response to one or more disease-modifying antirheumatic drugs. Etanercept is used in conjunction with more recognized therapies like methotrexate or alone as monotherapy. Allergic reactions to etanercept are rare, although itching or rash at the injection site may occur. The long-term effects of anti-TNF medications are not known, especially with the body's defense mechanisms against infection or malignancies. Patients who develop a new infection while undergoing treatment with etanercept should be monitored closely. Treatment should be discontinued in patients with serious infections. Other side effects occur infrequently, but include headache, nasal congestion, dizziness, sore throat, cough, generalized weakness, abdominal pain, rash, lung problems, shortness of breath, or inflammation of the sinuses.

Infliximab

Infliximab (Remicade) is a second antitumor therapy. Infliximab is a monoclonal antibody. This antibody was developed to accurately and specifically target tumor necrosis factor or TNF. Medical studies have shown that infliximab effectively relieves the signs and symptoms of RA with methotrexate.

Some people notice mild reactions like itching or a stinging feeling, and rarely chills, difficulty in breathing, or low blood pressure during the infusion. When reactions occur, they resolve if the infusion is stopped or temporarily slowed. Subsequent infusion reactions necessitate premedicating with acetaminophen or antihistamines. If no premedications are given, the patient can resume a normal schedule following the infusion.

Caution

All TNF blocking agents and concomitant immunosuppressive therapy alter the immune response, including the response to infection. Those individuals with chronic infections or a history of recurring infection should probably avoid anti-TNF treatment. There is a concern about inducing cancers, although clinically this has not been a problem. Blood tests are not routinely done to monitor therapy.

Other Treatments for Arthritis

More treatments exist for arthritis than you can imagine. While some treatments have scientific basis, some do not.

Skin Rubs

Many people with arthritis swear by the soothing qualities of topical creams, oils, gels, ointments, and sprays that can be applied directly to the skin over areas of tenderness or the joints themselves. Most of these medications are available over the counter at the pharmacy. The natural impulse to gently rub areas of soreness around a painful joint or muscle will bring comforting warmth to the area of tenderness. Home remedies have been used for years as rubs for the same reasons. They provide relief of pain and comforting warmth to the area. The wide variety of available rubs at the drugstore today offers invaluable temporary relief for some ailments—relief not provided by oral medications. Today's rubs contain a number of analgesics and other ingredients that are well absorbed into the skin. The massaging effect involved in applying the creams has a benefit all of its own. There is also a tremendous placebo effect.

The most common active ingredients include salicylates that have an important anti-inflammatory effect. Menthol, oil of wintergreen, camphor, and eucalyptus oil irritate the skin. Irritants stimulate the nerve endings and cause other feelings, which then mask the sensation of pain by distracting attention from the source of pain.

Some NSAIDs are available as creams or rubs and are absorbed through the skin.

Capsaicin is the substance in chili peppers that makes them hot. Over-the-counter creams that contain capsaicin reduce the sensation of pain by blocking the ability of the nerve endings around a joint to send pain impulses to the brain. Capsaicin creams are applied in small amounts directly on the skin over areas of pain three to four times a day. The pain will return once the cream is no longer applied. It can take a few weeks for the capsaicin to work. It is important to wash your hands after each application and keep the cream away from your eyes.

Antibiotics
A tetracycline antibiotic like minocycline has been shown to inhibit the enzymes metallaproteinases. Metallaproteinases degrade cartilage and harm the joint. Tetracycline is not currently approved by the FDA in the treatment of rheumatoid arthritis, yet many physicians use this medicine in an off-label fashion. "Off-label" implies that the drug or medication is approved by the FDA for at least one other illness, but it is being used in a different illness for which it has not been proven to date to help scientifically or statistically. Off-label use of medication is appropriate if the patient has been given an informed consent. An informed consent educates the patient to the off-label use and potential benefits versus risks, along with an explanation of accepted and recognized other treatments. The precise mechanism of action of tetracycline is unclear. Potential mechanisms of action might be its antimicrobial or antibiotic effect if infection is a cause of arthritis, or its effects on other portions of the immune system. Although early results in some studies are of interest, enthusiasm for tetracycline in the treatment of RA must be tempered. Additional studies must be completed and show favorable response before tetracycline can be recommended over current second-line agents in RA. Dizziness is the most commonly observed side effect. As with other tetracyclines, however, minocycline is potentially injurious to the liver.

Injections within the Joint
Injecting a swollen painful joint with intra-articular steroid preparations is usually effective and well tolerated. It is important that

the swollen joint is not infected. Results may be variable, but usually last for several days to months. Some steroids include triamcinolone hexacetonide (Aristospan) or triamcinolone diacetate (Aristocort). These preparations are insoluble and crystallize within the joint space. This allows most of the medicine to stay within the joint and minimize more systemic effects, although that still occurs. For example, injection of steroid medicine into one knee will usually help the other knee too. The same joint should not be injected more often than every three or four months or longer if possible. As a rule of thumb, it is not recommended to inject more than three large joints at any one setting. Even with insoluble steroid, systemic effects occur.

Arthrocentesis

One of the most beneficial and important tools available to the rheumatologist is the ability to remove fluid from a swollen joint or bursa with little discomfort to the patient.

Removal of fluid from an inflamed area provides comfort, especially if there is so much fluid that the area is tight or tense. Swelling stretches pain fibers and nerves. Unfortunately, fluid accumulates quickly if there is no other intervention to disrupt the cycle of events and the inflammation.

Aspiration or removal of the fluid is usually important to determine the characteristics of the fluid and the possibility of infection or other cause. Analysis under a special polarizing microscope can reveal crystals diagnostic of gout or pseudogout. Other crystals can also be discovered. The number of white cells helps classify the fluid as inflammatory or noninflammatory and helps sort out rheumatoid arthritis from osteoarthritis. Further examination in the laboratory can determine the presence of infection.

Only a few compounds are safely put within the joint. Over the years many medicines have been tried. Surgeons instill antibiotics within the joint or embed antibiotics in cement placed within the joint to fight infection. Several anesthetics are safely placed within the joint space. Their benefit is usually short-lived. Steroids placed within the joint are extremely helpful.

Hyaluronic acid (Hyalgan, Synvisc) is injected within the joint space weekly for three times. Hyaluronic acid is a natural viscoelastic agent found in the normal joint fluid. Joint fluid functions as a lubricant and shock absorber because of the hyaluronic acid. After the effects of arthritis, the joint accumulates more fluid, but the amount of hyaluronic acid diminishes. The joint fluid then loses its normal elasticity and viscosity properties and its ability to act as a shock absorber. Three injections restore the elastic and viscous nature of the fluid, lubricate the joint, and allow the fluid again to absorb the painful shocking motion of walking or running.

Pain is relieved for six to twelve months. Hyaluronic acid injections are indicated for the treatment of knee pain in osteoarthritis patients who have not responded adequately to conservative therapy or simple analgesic treatment. These injections are helpful in those individuals that are intolerant of therapies like NSAIDs, or those trying to delay surgery of the knee.

Vaccinations

Vaccinations to prevent infections are important to the arthritis patient. Vaccines play no role in treating arthritis otherwise. Inactivated vaccines use viruses or bacteria that cannot reproduce. These types of vaccines pose little risk or danger to immunocompromised arthritis patients because of their drug therapies, including steroids or cancer drugs. Vaccines that only alter viruses or bacteria are either attenuated or live. In individuals with a suppressed immune system, attenuated viruses could grow unchecked and result in infection. For these reasons, oral polio vaccine (OPV) should not be given to anyone in close contact with an immunosuppressed person, since the virus sheds from the vaccinated individual for as long as a month following vaccination. Other attenuated vaccines to avoid include varicella for chicken pox and measles, mumps, and rubella or MMR. Immunosuppressed individuals exposed to measles should receive gamma globulin shots.

- Tetanus-Diphtheria (TD) is given to everyone during his or her youth. A booster is given every ten years. Both tetanus and diphtheria are potentially serious infections prevented by vaccination.

- Hepatitis B vaccination is given in a series of three injections for several months, and should be administered to all young sexually active adults.

- Pneumococcal infection leads to serious problems. Everyone over sixty-five years of age should be vaccinated. Individuals with chronic disease or who have a condition like arthritis associated with an impaired immune system because of their illness or treatment should be vaccinated. Revaccination is given in the first five years. It is often given at the same time as the flu vaccination in our office.

- Influenza vaccine should be given to all individuals over sixty-five years of age and those with any chronic illness. Individuals allergic to eggs or egg products should avoid vaccines made from eggs.

- Lyme vaccine is relatively new. Two doses of vaccine raise immunity by fifty percent, and a third dose increases the protection to more than eighty percent. A booster immunization is suggested every two years. In areas where Lyme disease is common, it is recommended that nearly everyone who will be exposed to ticks through animals or outdoor activities be vaccinated.

Vaccinate

Individuals with chronic forms of arthritis and immunosuppression because of disease or drug therapy should have most of the above vaccines. The benefits far outweigh the risks. People with chronic forms of arthritis need the added protection. Attenuated vaccines need to be avoided.

Alternative Treatments

Alternative treatments are too numerous to list, but several deserve mentioning.

Acupuncture

The lack of good scientific studies is the reason that most of the medical establishment has not accepted acupuncture. However, the Chinese have accepted it for thousands of years. Acupuncture grew out of the concept of patterns of energy flow through the body that are essential to health; the idea that two complementary forces, either negative or positive, make up all aspects of life. When the forces are in balance the fundamental life force flows evenly through the body and results in good health. Traditional Chinese medicine believes you can regulate this flow with acupuncture needles by stimulating certain points of the body. Acupuncture involves the stimulation of anatomical locations on the skin by a variety of techniques. Stimulation of acupuncture points employs the penetration of the skin by thin, solid metallic needles that are manipulated manually or by electrical stimulation. Acupuncture is used by millions of American patients and performed by thousands of physicians.

Although evidence suggests that acupuncture causes physiologic changes in the body, Western medicine has neither proven nor accepted acupuncture. It is possible that the beneficial effects of acupuncture on arthritis are coming from an endorphin effect that abolishes pain, and from cortisol as a result of stimulation. Acupuncture stimulates the pituitary gland of the brain to secrete ACTH, which in turn stimulates the adrenal gland to secrete cortisol, the most potent anti-inflammatory known to man. One of the advantages of acupuncture is that the incidence of adverse effects is substantially lower than with many drugs or other accepted medical procedures used for the same condition. However, there may be an occurrence of adverse events in the practice of acupuncture, some of which are life-threatening.

For any therapeutic intervention, there can be a "nonspecific" effect that accounts for a substantial proportion of its effectiveness, and thus should not be casually discounted, including the quality of the relationship between the patient and doctor, the expectations of the patient, and the belief systems of the doctor and patient.

Unfortunately, acupuncture does not lend itself well to completing a double-blinded study to determine its effectiveness. Many insurance companies cover the expense of acupuncture, perhaps because of the diversity of our population. Some states have even mandated insurance coverage and its use appears to be on an increase.

Chiropractic Treatment

Chiropractic treatment, perceived as satisfactory by many, is relatively low in cost, and facilitates return to work for many afterwork injuries. It is applied principally to musculoskeletal disorders, especially spinal problems and injuries. The modern science of chiropractic therapy includes spinal manipulation. Chiropractic treatment differs from conventional medicine in that it discourages drug therapy and surgery, and instead, it is based on the body's ability to heal itself. Chiropractors remove or correct malalignments of the spine or subluxations by spinal manipulation or adjustments. Chiropractors often give advice about diet, nutrition, and exercise. Spinal manipulation is probably somewhat an effective symptomatic therapy for some patients with acute low back pain. The efficacy of spinal manipulation and the cost effectiveness of chiropractic treatment relative to other care is controversial. The use of cervical manipulation arouses the greatest concern about safety and injury to the patient. Physicians generally accept the role of chiropractic medicine in treating selected musculoskeletal conditions, but oppose its use in other systemic diseases like hypertension, asthma, or most systemic forms of arthritis.

Holistic Medicine

Holistic practices provide attention and gives care in relation to body, mind, and spirit. There is no proof of efficacy, effectiveness of cost, or validity. The cornerstone is the concept that the whole is made up of interdependent parts. Therefore, what happens to us physically, mentally, emotionally, or spiritually will impact all other aspects of who we are as individuals. When possible, treatments are selected that support the body's natural healing system.

Homeopathy

Homeopathy provides numerous remedies prepared from plants. The safety and symbolism are especially appealing. Naturopathy employs a selection of counseling, diet and nutritional advice, herbal medicine, homeopathy, exercises, massage and manipulation.

Osteopathy

Osteopaths have a complete range of manipulative techniques characterized by minimum force and greatest specificity. Osteo-paths claim specific patterns of spinal dysfunction correlate to internal organ problems. Many osteopaths have the same privileges to practice medicine as licensed medical doctors.

Stress Reduction

Acupressure, shiatsu, and reflexology are claimed to reduce stress. They are applied in a variety of minor musculoskeletal complaints. Pain can be relieved with relaxation therapy, biofeedback, meditation, counseling, and hypnotherapy.

Balneopathy

Water therapy is appealing and effective in the treatment of arthritis pain. Buoyancy is useful and easy on the joints. Mudpacks and mineral therapy are partially beneficial. The chemical content of the water is of questionable significance. This treatment form is especially popular in Eastern Europe.

Diets

Many naturopaths and other proponents of alternative treatments suggest fasting, often as part of a treatment program for arthritis. There is no scientific research to justify treatments like purgation, intestinal antisepsis, or colonic irrigation. Unfortunately, these treatments rely on gullibility. Other dietary advice from alternative practitioners ranges from good sound nutritional princi- ples to fads, myths, and quackery. Diets rich in fish oils are often recommended and have some theoretical basis, as do many unproven remedies.

> *The leap from science to effectiveness is, however, a big jump.*

Reduction of obesity, adequate nutrition, eating from all the major food groups is good advice. Vitamin supplements are useful but large doses have no proven definite ther- apeutic efficacy.

Unproven Remedies

Billions of dollars are spent every year on unproven arthritis treatments. Although proven treatments take time to work, at least their safety and effectiveness have been well documented in repeated rigidly controlled scientific studies. Unproven remedies, such as bee venom and large doses of vitamins, are treatments that have not been shown to work by repeated scientific studies. All their side effects are unknown.

> *If a treatment sounds too good, has a secret formula, or fails to list all its contents, be suspicious and avoid it.*

It has been suggested that fish oils lessen the inflammation of arthritis and its symptoms. Fish oils interfere with the process of inflam- mation. Fish oils contain substances called omege-3-fatty acids that reduce the body's production of another substance called arachidonic acid. The breakdown products of arachidonic acid result in a series of other substances that are very important as media- tors of inflammation. Anything that reduces these substances may have a positive effect on the inflammation associated with arthri- tis. Arachidonic acid is formed from fatty ac- ids in a normal diet, but omega-3-fatty acids in fish oil are different. These fish oils taken in a normal diet can prevent the body from making arachidonic acid and thus inhibit painful inflammation. Although some stud- ies have proven this correct, so far the bene- fits are very small and are not worth the ef- fort. Initial studies utilized large quantities of fish oils, much more than what any normal diet consumes. Cod liver oil does contain small amounts of the fatty acids found in fish oil supplement, but huge amounts are still necessary to match the amounts used in re- search studies. Cod liver oil also contains some vitamins in large amounts that are ex- cessive and detrimental for other reasons.

Other popular unproven remedies include copper bracelets, horse liniment (DMSO), sitting in uranium mines, vibrators, and spe- cial diets. A number of clinics have been es- tablished just on the basis of unproven reme- dies. Promoters of unproven remedies abound and tend to make exaggerated claims. There is no proven remedy that will cure arthritis, be effective in all forms of arthritis, or is beneficial just because it is natural. In addition, most of these remedies are expensive and somewhat unusual. Testimonials are very limited and do not necessarily correlate to all people.

Two recent unproven remedies include the nutritional supplements glucosamine sulphate and chondroitin sulfate. These two substances are suggested as natural remedies to cure arthritis. Studies done on these substances do not appear to meet the stringent requirements of a well-conducted clinical trial. These criteria include sufficient numbers of similar patients under similar circumstances in a double-blinded fashion over a sufficient duration of time by reputable investigators.

So far, these substances appear to be more of a marketing success than treatment for any form of arthritis.

Both compounds are the subject of a bestseller. Proponents suggest these nutrients bolster cartilage by stimulating new cartilage growth and inhibiting naturally occurring enzymes that destroy cartilage. These supplements are readily available at health food stores and are not regulated by the FDA. Characterizing these supplements as a cure on television talk shows or books without additional proof of results from testing is irresponsible. It is important that people taking these supplements not stop taking their conventional therapies. In our clinic, no serious harm has been seen with these compounds, but neither has any patient had a significant benefit. At best, these supplements are comparable to modest anti-inflammatories, but without the ability to rebuild cartilage or modify the joint.

Medical Marijuana

In some states, medical marijuana is permitted to relieve symptoms of serious conditions like arthritis. Because of marijuana's psychoactive effects, its acceptance for medical benefit has been slow and resistive. Its ability to relieve the nausea, vomiting, or loss of appetite associated with the chemotherapy of cancer or AIDS is well accepted. There may be benefits on glaucoma. Marijuana's active ingredients are called cannabinoids, and can suppress the pain of arthritis and possibly the inflammation. Currently scientists are exploring different ways to deliver the active ingredient in some other form than smoking and its associated toxicity. Although many doctors believe in the benefits of medical marijuana, others are skeptical that the legalization of marijuana may be a ploy for those who want legalization for recreational use.

Arthritis Is Chronic and Incurable

The fact that most arthritis is chronic and incurable leaves the door open for a number of unproven remedies. Comparison of arthritis by individuals with different disease or anecdotal stories will abound. Unproven remedies will continue to drive up the cost of health care, create false hope for some individuals, and for some have them leave behind conventional medical care that isn't perfect, but which has helped the majority of patients with arthritis.

The key to success against unproven remedies is to be well educated: check with your doctor, be skeptical, ask questions, realize that just because it is in writing doesn't mean that it is proven, and finally, look for ingredients and recognized treatments that have stood up to the test of time.

Herbs

Herbs are used by one third of the adult American population today. People are turning to untraditional sources to alleviate or prevent symptoms produced by a number of illnesses, including arthritis. Users proclaim herbal remedies are natural and make them feel better, and have milder and fewer side effects than other available medications or over-the-counter remedies. Herbal supplement sales have more than doubled in the past decade. Giant pharmaceutical companies are also becoming involved. At least some of this popularity is motivated by consumer demand for different ways to maintain health. Deregulation of the herbal industry allows manufacturers to make product claims on labels without first getting them approved by the Food and Drug Administration (FDA). Prior to deregulation, lengthy clinical trials had to be completed that were time-consuming and expensive. The FDA requires that herbal supplements list all plants and chemicals contained in them on the label.

The ground swell of American interest in herbal remedies is curious, since herbs have been widely used in Asian cultures for thousands of years. Even modern Europe has a long tradition of honoring herbal remedies. By contrast, the United States has lagged behind. Today, at least part of the aging population of America has become disenchanted with Western medicine and seeks out more control over their health.

Herbal medicine may be just what the doctor ordered.

Conventional medicine is often perceived as cold and remote or synthetic, compared to the natural substances of herbal preparations. Of course, the active ingredient of an herb is a chemical. If the doctor is inaccessible, the clerk at the health food store is not. A rediscovery of the healing powers of plants only marks a return to an ancient form of medicine still used by the majority of the world's population. Many current modern medicines are derived from herbs, including aspirin, which is from white willow bark.

Herbs are far less potent than pharmaceuticals and therefore are less toxic. They possess far less side effects. Our diversity of cultures may also explain the increased use of herbal medicines. Despite the questionable efficacy and benefits of herbs, especially with regard to arthritis, the medicinal use of these will most likely continue.

Consumers spent more than twelve billion dollars on natural supplements last year, and sales continue to grow. Even so-called functional foods now contain herbal remedies to perk you up, and others to calm you down. Fashionable soda drinks now contain herbal supplements. Americans make more visits to nontraditional physicians than to their family doctors. The rapid expansion of herbal medicines comes at some risk for the American consumer. None of these products are regulated as well as over-the-counter medications or foods. When you open the bottle of a nutritional supplement, you really do not know what's in it.

Few rheumatologists have received formal training in nutrition and herbal medicines. Because of consumer interest, the medical profession is responding with more than fifty percent of medical schools now offering courses in unconventional medicine.

The effectiveness of many treatments may be the result of placebo or the patient's desire to believe in a cure and this having an influence on well-being. Unfortunately, the history of dietary supplements has on occasion caused untoward results.

HERBAL SUPPLEMENTS PROPOSED BENEFITS

Echinacea

- Boosts the immune system and fights colds

Ginseng

- Increases stamina and endurance

Ginkgo

- Slows the effects of dementia, increases circulation

Saw Palmetto

- Slows prostate disease

Goldenseal

- Helps sore throats, stomach ulcers, hemorrhoids, canker sores

Garlic

- Reduces high blood pressure

Evening Primrose

- Helps GI disorders, asthma, PMS, psoriasis, and arthritis

St. John's Wort

- Helps depression

Kava Kava

- Helps anxiety

Milk Thistle

- Helps protect the liver

Bilberry

- Helps eye disorders

Ginger Root

- Relieves pain associated with osteoarthritis

CHAPTER 31

Menopause

Menopause affects a woman's response to her arthritis and other treatments. All postmenopausal women should consider estrogen replacement therapy (ERT). Estrogen is a female hormone produced by the ovaries. Treatment replaces the estrogen that is no longer naturally produced by the body after menopause. Estrogen is usually taken by itself, but in some people must be combined with a progestin, a synthetic form of progesterone. Progesterone is another female hormone. Hormone therapy can relieve many of the symptoms associated with menopause, including hot flashes and vaginal dryness. Long-term hormone therapy provides two important other benefits, including protection against coronary heart disease and protection against osteoporosis. Coronary heart disease is the leading cause of death among postmenopausal women and osteoporosis is the most common cause for fracture. Estrogen therapy decreases the risk for hip fracture.

Side Effects

Women who take estrogen alone over many years are at a greater risk for developing endometrial cancer. Endometrial cancer occurs in the uterine lining. This type of cancer is easily detected early and generally requires a hysterectomy. Combination therapy with a progestin and estrogen eliminates the risk for cancer caused by taking estrogen alone in a woman who still has her uterus. Women who take estrogen for many years may also be at risk for developing breast cancer. The degree of risk remains controversial among experts in the field. Other side effects such as bloating, breast tenderness, headache or irritability are usually mild and resolve after a few months of therapy. These symptoms result in some women's intolerance to ERT. Menstrual spotting sometimes occurs while taking hormones, and results in confusion about the occurrence of endometrial cancer. This requires the need for endometrial monitoring or the removal of a small amount of tissue from within the uterus.

The decision to take long-term hormone therapy is a complex one. In those women who have had a hysterectomy and need ERT, there does not appear to be a reason to add a progestin. It would be impossible to develop uterine cancer without a uterus. If an individual is at an increased risk for breast cancer, the risk of hormonal therapy may outweigh its benefits. In women with no particular risk factors for cancer and who do not have a uterus, treatment with estrogen alone is acceptable. If the uterus is present, therapy with estrogen and a progestin eliminates the risk for uterine cancer. The best course of action in the future is unclear and will require further studies for clarification.

Designer Hormones

An alternative to traditional hormones for postmenopausal women is raloxifene (Evista). This is a selective estrogen receptor modulator (SERM). Evista activates specific estrogen receptors, while it does not activate others. Therefore, it has estrogen-like effects on bone and increases bone mineral density, but to a lesser extent than estrogen, and on lipid decreases metabolism. Most importantly, Evista lacks estrogen-like effects on breast and uterine tissue. Without that effect, it does not cause breast tenderness or vaginal bleeding, does not increase the risk of breast or uterine cancer in early studies so far, and does not require concomitant progesterone treatment if a woman still has her uterus. Side effects of the therapy are minimal, but do include increased blood clotting problems, hot flashes, and leg cramps. These medications do not treat the vasomotor symptoms or hot flashes of menopause.

Menopause signals the beginning of a new phase in a woman's life, a time when risk for osteoporosis begins to increase dramatically.

New SERMs are expected in the near future.

Generic Drugs

Generic drugs generally cost less than brand-name drugs. As managed health care becomes more prevalent, more health plans are requiring the substitution of brand-name drugs with generic drugs. This is important for individuals with arthritis who take medications for extended periods of time. For example, saving twenty dollars a month for one drug would add up to two hundred and forty dollars a year.

The question of course is whether generic drugs are at a cost to your health.

Definition of Generics

A generic drug is a copy of a brand-name drug that is developed and marketed by a pharmaceutical drug company other than the original company that discovered the compound. Major companies spend an average of ten years or more and five hundred million dollars to develop a new drug and bring it to market. For at least a while, the pharmaceutical company receives a patent to protect its ownership and exclusivity of a new chemical formulation. A portion of the time granted includes the years in research. This diminishes the time in years that a company may recoup costs and make a profit later when the drug is marketed. For these reasons, the usefulness to the company that did all the research is relatively short. If you add launching and marketing costs, new drugs are the most expensive ones available.

Once the patent expires, other pharmaceutical companies can produce and sell the same drug, usually at a much-reduced cost. They do not have the start up costs like the other company, including the research and development costs. These savings can be passed on to the consumer.

Standards of Generic Medicine

In 1984, the FDA instituted standards requiring generic drugs to have the same active ingredients, dosage breakdowns, strengths, and forms, as their brand-name counterparts. The generic manufacturer must prove and demonstrate the generic drug has the same bioequivalence or acts on the body in the same way as the brand-name drugs. "Equivalent to" is not necessarily the same as "equal to." The law allows a ten-to-twenty-percent variation in bioequivalence. Most generic drugs do not vary from the brand-name equivalents more than five percent. Instances in which generic drugs do not work as well as brand-name equivalents have been rare.

The primary variation between generic and brand-name drugs is in the fillers and binders that affect the look and taste of the drug to hold it together. The FDA requires that all drugs be safe and effective. Since generic drugs have the same active ingredients and work the same way in the body, they should be safe and effective.

The FDA allows no drug to be made in substandard facilities. The same manufacturing practices and requirements apply to both generic and brand-name drugs. Many generic drugs are actually manufactured by brand-name manufacturers. The converse is also true: generic manufacturers often produce brand-name products.

With that information in mind, there is probably no reason to avoid generics. Although generics are not the best choice for all people in all situations, the cost savings they offer make it possible for more people to afford treatment.

Cost of Medicine

Rising health-care costs continue to be a source of great national concern and debate. There has been interest over the costs of

NSAIDs and their contribution to total health-care costs. In 1991, prescription drugs accounted for approximately thirty-six billion dollars or five percent of total health-care costs. This however, greatly underestimates the contribution of NSAID costs to health care. It does not include the total costs of treating patients with these medications. Retail prices have been a major focus of attention. The total costs of therapy with NSAIDs include not only the price of the drug, but also the costs of monitoring patients for potential toxicities when they occur or paying for concomitant protective medicines like acid-blocking agents. Drug monitoring and toxicity costs represent major components of total medication costs, particularly for patients with chronic arthritic diseases for whom medications are an important element of their health care and who need to take medications on a long-term basis.

Package Insert

The package insert is the FDA-approved product labeling for a particular medication and is the best and most reliable source of information, particularly about the safety of a drug that is readily available to consumers. Unfortunately, the information is written for doctors and pharmacists and is difficult to interpret. Specific sections of the insert are still useful, including indications and usage, contraindications, adverse reactions, drug interactions, and dosage and administration. All of this same information is found in the Physician's Desk Reference or PDR. This information is available for both branded medications and generics.

Direct-to-Consumer Advertising

Direct-to-consumer (DTC) advertising is relatively new, but is occurring at an increasing rate, both in print and in broadcast advertising. The drug companies are increasingly advertising their products directly to consumers. Recent advertising budgets for this kind of advertising have exceeded over 1.5 billion dollars. However, the drug companies still spend most of their budget of over 5 billion dollars for advertising on doctors. The FDA is responsible for the monitoring of this advertising and the protection of the public from serious consequences of false and misleading prescription drug advertising. Newspaper and magazine articles are also a form of DTC advertising.

Typically, the newer drugs expected to be major blockbusters for the drug companies and utilized by millions of Americans are the ones advertised. Advertisements play an important role in educating the public. DTC advertising is required by law to provide disclaimers about prescribing information for a particular drug, including precautions and possible side effects.

Lab Tests

Laboratory tests are necessary to make the diagnosis of arthritis. Blood tests help confirm the diagnosis, monitor therapy, and look for serious consequences of the disease or treatment.

- *Antinuclear Antibody (ANA)* This marker for autoimmunity is found in over ninety-five percent of those individuals with established and diagnosed systemic lupus erythematosus (SLE), but it is also found in a number of other closely related illnesses including Sjögren's syndrome, rheumatoid arthritis, polymyositis, mixed connective tissue disease, and scleroderma.

There are a number of normal individuals without any evidence of arthritis or collagen vascular disease, who have a positive ANA in their blood sample.

The frequency of finding a positive ANA test in healthy people approaches thirty percent. ANAs are more common in the elderly and in women. The titers are usually low. Relatives of patients with disorders associated with ANAs appear to be at a substantially increased risk for the development of these antibodies. The reason for this is unknown, but genetic factors may play a role.

Specific autoantibodies within the ANA can be demonstrated and help sort out different subsets of disease. The strength of the positivity of the test is reported as a titer. Blood is first tested slightly diluted, then tested repeatedly over again in greater dilutions. The greater the dilution of the blood done while doing the test results in a higher titer result. This usually has more clinical significance and importance. Normal individuals with positive ANAs usually have low titers. The methodology of the test also provides a visual pattern that is more specific for different subsets of disease. Repeated tests are not helpful in monitoring disease activity. At least five percent of the population is estimated to have autoantibodies without systemic disease or medical problems. Although these antibodies reflect a specific type of reaction, their presence is not indicative of ongoing harm or damage to the body. Once established, these antibodies persist for years.

The ANA screen is the most sensitive test used in diagnosing lupus. The positive ANA is useful when the diagnosis is unclear, but two or three other features of lupus exist. Just using ANA testing to screen for lupus is undesirable.

- *Rheumatoid Factor (RF)* This test is positive in about seventy-five percent of those patients with the definite diagnosis of rheumatoid arthritis. This test is of prognostic value. Individuals with a positive test usually have more severe disease, especially if high-titered. The RF correlates well with the presence of nodules at the elbows, erosions on x-ray, and decreases slightly after treatment. A positive RF will most likely not become negative later. The RF isn't useful in monitoring activity of disease.

- *HLA-B27* This test measures a specific genetic marker in the blood that has been associated with a number of diseases, especially ankylosing spondylitis or Reiter's syndrome. It occurs in over ninety percent of these patients, especially if the sacroiliac joints are involved with the arthritis. Six percent of the normal population also has the presence of this genetic marker. This marker does not necessarily indicate that disease exists. Genetic markers do not change over time or with activity of disease. Genetic markers are not useful in monitoring disease activity.

- *Erythrocyte Sedimentation Rate (ESR)* This blood test correlates to the activity of arthritis and is useful to monitor response to treatment. It is a nonspecific test of inflammation. The test may be elevated in other conditions like cancer, infection, or other disease. On occasion, even in the presence of a severely swollen joint the ESR is normal, however most of the time the greater amount of inflammation, the higher the test result. The test is done by several different methods, usually takes a full one hour to interpret, is done in a simple office laboratory, and is relatively inexpensive.

- *Muscle Enzymes (CPK, Aldolase)* Inflamed muscle cells swell and rupture releasing their contents into the bloodstream. CPK and aldolase are important muscle enzymes that are within the muscle cell. Dying muscle cells release enzymes every day into the blood, which are easily measured. Normal levels within the blood are established. During inflammatory muscle disease or injury to the muscle cell, the muscle enzyme levels are hundreds of times greater than normal. Muscle enzyme levels decrease in response to treatment.

- *Complete Blood Count (CBC)* This test is utilized by all practicing physicians and is abnormal in several rheumatic illnesses. The CBC measures the red cell count that carries oxygen, the white cell count that helps measure the ability to fight infection, and the platelets that help plug up blood vessels and prevent bleeding. Anemia or a low red cell count is the most common laboratory manifestation of rheumatoid arthritis. Anemia can be evidence of gastrointestinal bleeding from stomach ulcers. Checking the stool for occult blood examines for evidence of possible gastrointestinal (GI) blood loss. Iron studies help distinguish the cause of anemia too.

- *Biopsy* Biopsies of skin, muscle, or other tissue provide important information and help with the diagnosis. In rheumatic illnesses for example, looking for inflamed blood vessels in tissues provides evidence of vasculitis. A temporal artery biopsy will demonstrate vasculitis in temporal arteritis if it is present. Some biopsies require special expertise and handling. Muscle biopsies require special technologies and staining during examination.

- *Electromyography (EMG), Nerve Conduction Velocities (NCV)* These electrodiagnostic tests help identify pressure on nerves or inflammation of muscles. Localization of the area of inflammation in muscle helps identify which muscle will most likely show diagnostic changes on biopsy. EMGs are helpful in identifying nerve root impingement like sciatica.

NCVs identify pressure on the median nerve in carpal tunnel syndrome. Occasionally, systemic rheumatic illnesses affect several nerves of the hands or feet at the same time. Identification on EMG can diagnose a neuropathy or neuritis.

- *Complement Studies* Complement is a protein in the blood that amplifies the immune system. During the immune process and inflammation, complement is consumed and when measured in the blood is low. Low complement levels in the blood are an indirect measure of disease activity.

- *Antinuclearanticytoplasmic Antibodies (C-ANCA or P-ANCA)* These antibodies are often a sign of active disease, especially vasculitis. They are commonly measured in Wegener's granulomatosis.

- *Hepatitis Testing* There are a number of markers for all of the forms of hepatitis. Hepatitis B is associated with vasculitis. Hepatitis C has several musculoskeletal manifestations.

- *Synovial Fluid Analysis* Tests are done on specimens taken directly from a swollen joint space or bursa. The synovial fluid is examined under a microscope and cultured in the laboratory for infection. With the help of a special polarizing microscope uric acid crystals can be demon-strated and confirm the diagnosis of gout. The characteristics of the crystals differentiate gout from a similar crystal-induced arthritis like pseudogout. Increased white cells in the fluid suggest an inflammatory state and differentiate arthritis like RA from OA or infection. A low level of glucose in the joint fluid as compared to the blood suggests infection. Just removing joint fluid alone relieves pressure and pain in the joint. Unfortunately, without further intervention, the relief is usually short-lived and fluid reaccummulates quickly.

- *Routine Blood Tests* Routine blood tests are done to determine the metabolic status of an individual and include electrolytes like sodium and potassium, liver function tests like enzymes and bilirubin, kidney function tests, blood glucose for diabetes, protein levels in the blood, and calcium levels. These tests are included in all inclusive panels. As Medicare requirements get stricter, many of these panels have become more specific with regards to organ function or disease, and are called metabolic panels, hepatic panels, or liver panels.

- *Radiology* Plain radiographs or x-rays are used for several reasons. A chest x-ray is used to determine the size of the heart, the possibility of fluid accumulation around the heart secondary to pericarditis, and the clarity of the lung fields. The lung fields can reveal infection, pneumonia, or fluid. The list of problems determined by a chest x-ray is long. This remains an important initial screening tool to determine the status of the heart and lungs. X-rays of joints help determine alignment, deformity, bone density, or arthritis. Weight-bearing knee x-rays will show the amount of cartilage that remains between the two major bones of that joint. X-rays do not show soft tissues well. Magnetic resonance images (MRI) or computerized tomography (CT) will delineate soft tissues like nerves, tumors, or collections of fluid. Ultrasound is a useful and simple radiological technique to look at blood vessels or organ size and function throughout the body. Ultrasound can identify popliteal cysts of the knee. Arteriograms inject dye into the blood vessels and outline the vessel's course and diameter.

Clinical Drug Trials

Clinical drug trials allow new medications to be tried in the treatment of arthritis. The drug therapy for arthritis has no magical pill or cure. Neither is there any special drug therapy, herbal medicine, surgery, dietary supplement, or other therapy that is clearly more advantageous than all the rest. Physician experts such as rheumatologists appear to favor drug therapy, with the judicious use of other interventions interspersed among them. Other interventions include hydrotherapy, stress reduction, and even acupuncture for pain control. There are several reasons for the utilization of medications. Historically medications work, at least to some degree, and drugs make sense with the current degree of our knowledge and understanding of the disease processes in arthritis. Most current research for new medicines is done in the United States by pharmaceutical companies. Together these companies continue to invest billions of dollars a year, more than the entire federal budget for the National Institutes of Health, the American premier health research institute. Of all the drugs approved by the Food and Drug Administration (FDA) from 1981 to 1990, over ninety percent were discovered by pharmaceutical industry scientists, less than ten percent at universities in the United States and other labs, and only one percent at government labs.

The Wealth of Medical Information

The pharmaceutical companies have obvious reasons for making such commitments. The challenges of finding a cure or relief to chronic diseases are greater than ever before; so is the scientific knowledge and technical resources at our disposal.

The wealth of information about disease process doubles every few years.

There is a huge market and need for new medicine both in the U.S. and in the world. Patients and families insist that we continue to explore new medicines to find cures that will make a difference for those individuals that have developed one of the more than 100 different forms of arthritis. New science has opened up bits of information and knowledge never previously understood. We have opportunities to treat diseases differently than ever before. Rather than just understanding the consequence of arthritis, we

now have a better understanding of the mechanisms of disease at a cellular level and even within the cell or intracellular level. We now have knowledge we did not understand just a few years ago. America has been more successful than any other country in providing the right mix of incentives to keep research moving forward. Nearly one half of the world-class drugs introduced over the past two decades came from the laboratories of American companies. No other country even came close. In other words, drug research is big business driven by the needs of patients, researchers, scientists, and investors. The financial expense of this research has been tremendous, but the rewards will be even greater.

The pharmaceutical companies have established large laboratories and research teams throughout the world. New super-computing and technologies enable them to screen hundreds of compounds and to patent them immediately. Based on the knowledge of disease, drugs can now be designed and built molecule by molecule to interact at a cellular level specific for a disease state. This process takes considerable time and expense. Initial testing is confined to the laboratory and the test tube. Eventually, it must be tried in live animal experiments. This preclinical testing will characterize the effects of the drugs on models of the disease. There has been criticism of animal experimentation, yet it enables researchers to at least predict some of the effects in humans. A major difficulty is finding animal models that mimic human disease. Results are very different in animals than in humans. If testing is successful, the pharmaceutical company then asks the FDA for permission for further experimentation. The preclinical results are submitted and reviewed first by the FDA. At that time, the company requests an Investigational New Drug Application Approval (INDA) to begin testing in humans. If the FDA is satisfied with the review and decides that the potential benefits of testing in humans outweighs the risks involved, the stage is set for clinical trials.

All clinical drug trials must be approved by an Institutional Review Board (IRB). IRBs review the ethics and appropriateness of human experimentation. There are many of these at hospitals, universities, or other areas around the country. IRBs exist to protect the patient during human experimentation and consist of a cross section of individuals including scientists, medical doctors, pharmacists, nurses, clergy, and other people from the community. Essentially, the IRB reviews the study protocol, the patient's informed consent, the investigator and site, and the progress of the study to determine that the risks are reasonable in relation to the potential benefits. These built-in safeguards are designed to protect patients and their rights, and to prevent misleading promises or outcomes.

Phases of Clinical Trials

Clinical trials of experimental drugs in humans are done in three phases. Each successive phase involves a larger number of volunteer subjects. Even after a drug is released, clinical trials continue.

Clinical drug trials are double-blinded. Neither the patient, nor the doctor knows who is receiving the new medicine or the placebo.

The Challenge

Pharmaceutical research is a complex and challenging process. It may be met with failure at any stage. Of the thousands of compounds synthesized annually at major pharmaceutical companies, only a few will make it to a developmental stage and of these only a few will make it through a process that can take as much as a decade and cost an average of $500 million for each new drug that emerges from a company's pipeline. As with other inventions and discoveries, new chemical compounds with the potential to become medicines are protected by patent laws that grant inventors exclusive rights. After the patent expires, the invention passes to the public domain, the world of generic medicines. U.S. patent rights are traditionally granted for seventeen years from the date of grant. Additional research eventually shortens the remaining useful life of a patent to six or seven years once a new drug reaches

PHASES OF CLINICAL DRUG TRIALS

- **Phase I Clinical Trials** focus primarily on safety, and gather preliminary data on the effectiveness of a new compound. A wide range of doses of the compound are usually administered to a small group of healthy volunteers under close supervision. This is often in a hospital or in a rigidly controlled setting.

- **Phase II Clinical Trials** last longer and focus on the compound's safety and effectiveness against the illness it was orginally designed to treat. Strict guidelines for informed consent are observed so that the potential benefits and risks are clearly explained to the patients. Some of the patients will receive a placebo. Placebos are sugar pills that have no active ingredients.

- **Phase III Clinical Trials** are the final stage. Researchers confirm the results of earlier tests in large geographical patient populations. This takes several years and includes up to several thousand patients. Large geographically diverse groups are sought to eliminate the effects of possible unique genetic characteristics of patient populations, or local events that could alter drug response or monitoring, for example an outbreak of hepatitis in one community.

- **Phase IV Clinical Trials** occur after FDA approval of the medication. Even after the drug has received FDA approval after the New Drug Application (NDA) process, companies will continue to conduct post-marketing studies to monitor safety issues.

the marketplace. It is during this time that the pharmaceutical company must recover the enormous expense of research and development.

Clinical trials are usually conducted, but not limited to large metropolitan areas or university centers. However, private clinicians often contribute significantly to such research. Recruitment can sometimes be difficult at a university. Private physicians have access to large number of patients with established disease. Patient populations in large teaching institutions have already often participated in clinical trials. Physicians-in-training often lack the experience necessary to do studies, do not have access to many patients, and do not have the advantage of following the same patient during the length of the study.

Should You Volunteer for a Clinical Drug Trial?
Only patients who wish to participate in a clinical drug trial should. It should be entirely voluntary and treatment should not be

based just on willingness to participate. A volunteer is permitted to quit the study at any time, although in fairness to the study and its success, at the time of initiation of the study, a well-informed volunteer should be committed to finish the study as long as they know the benefits and risks. Even after signing an informed consent, a patient can leave the trial at any time and receive other conventional medical care without penalty. The informed consent must be read and signed before any study-related procedure or other action occurs. In addition, the investigator should explain the informed consent in detail and answer any and all questions the volunteer asks. An informed consent should leave the volunteer with an understanding of the protocol including the number of visits and procedures, previous studies with the medicine to date and known side effects, and importantly, other alternative, standard, or recognized treatments available.

Patients in clinical drug trials are among the first to receive the benefits of new research before it is widely available to others. However, just as the effects of standard treatments can't be entirely predicted, neither can the results of an experimental treatment.

Participants in clinical drug trials are monitored closely according to the strict guidelines of the protocol. Their participation becomes part of a larger project carried out in many areas and by many investigators who can then pool their ideas and results. It is hoped then that the knowledge gained is shared to the benefit of all patients with the same illness.

To determine the appropriateness of entering a clinical drug trial, a patient has a number of issues to consider. Some illnesses cause symptoms and even death unrelated to treatment. Therefore, unavoidable risks of the disease must be weighed against the benefits and risks of the new research treatment. Even standard treatments cannot predict guaranteed results or the absence of side effects. The demands of some studies can be significant for some patients who already do not feel well, although the new therapy has the potential to help. If a patient receives a placebo, there may be no benefit at all and the disease worsens with precious time lost. For some individuals with limited resources, clinical trials provide an opportunity to access health care or a specialist knowledgeable of their illness, and opportunities for further care, or directions after the study.

The myths and fears of clinical drug studies and human experimentation can be frightening. Some individuals will think of themselves as "guinea pigs in the laboratory." These ideas result from the fear of the unknown. It is imperative that the patient understand the informed consent and that anxieties are eased. During a research study, monitoring and observation is meticulous. It is believed that study patients actually receive better care than do patients receiving conventional care. If during a study it is clear that the treatment being received is not in the best interests of the patient, the patient should be discontinued from the study.

Resources

- Arthritis Foundation
  P.O. Box 1900
  Atlanta, Georgia 30326
  (800) 283-7800

- Food and Drug Administration
  5600 Fishers Lane
  Rockville, Maryland 20857
  (301) 443-3170

- National Osteoporosis Foundation
  1150 17th Street, Suite 500, N.W.
  Washington, D.C. 20036-4603

- Spondylitis Association of America
  P.O. Box 5872
  Sherman Oaks, California 91413
  (800) 777-8189

- Scleroderma Foundation
  89 Newbury Street, Suite 201
  Danvers, Massachusetts 01923
  (800) 722-HOPE (4673)
  (978) 750-4499
  Fax (978) 750-9902
  SFinfo@scleroderma.org

- Sjögren's Syndrome Foundation
  333 North Broadway
  Jerricho, New York 11753
  (800) 475-6473
  www.sjogrens.com

- National Sjögren's Syndrome Association
  5815 N. Black Canyon, Suite 103
  Phoenix, Arizona 85015-2200
  (602) 433-9844
  (800) 396-NSSA (6772)
  www.sjogrens.org

- American Lyme Disease Foundation, Inc.
  293 Route 100
  Somera, New York 10589
  (914) 277-6970

- Fibromyalgia Network
  P.O. Box 31750
  Tucson, Arizona 85751

- National Psoriasis Foundation
  6600 SW 92nd Avenue, Suite 300
  Portland, Oregon 97223

Index

A

acetaminophen 28, 55, 100, 120, 158, 172

activities of daily living (ADL) 133, 140

Actonel 18, 65, 145

acupressure 181

acupuncture 179–180, 201

adhesive capsulitis 9, 88, 115

adrenal suppression 143

AIDS 22, 72, 75, 153, 183

aldolase 59, 197

alendronate 18, 65, 145

allopurinol 37–38

American College of Rheumatology (ACR) xvi, 23, 32, 95, 122

Americans with Disabilities Act (ADA) 102

amitriptyline 33

analgesics 5, 40, 55, 87, 118, 120, 173

anemia 14, 22, 24–25, 64–65, 72, 122, 168, 197

ankle 2, 10, 26, 36, 44, 78, 138

ankylosing spondylitis 4, 41–42, 84, 86, 196

anticardiolipin antibodies 94, 111

antidepressants 33–34

anti-DNA antibody 25

antigens xvii, 22, 25, 61

antimalarials 28–29, 43, 91, 111, 121, 148–150, 152

antinuclear antibody (ANA) 3, 23–25, 29, 58, 195–196

antinuclearanticytoplasmic antibodies 198

antiphospholipid syndrome 24, 27, 93–94

arachidonic acid 182

Aralen 149

Arava 121, 148, 156

Aristocort 175

Aristospan 175

arthralgia 23, 75, 95

arthritis
    extra-articular 14, 122
    migratory 45
    mutilans 8, 43
    reactive 43, 71, 75
    rheumatoid (RA) xviii, 2–3, 7–9, 11–14, 23, 29, 34, 39, 41, 43–45, 49, 52, 54–55, 65, 68, 73–74, 78–80, 86–88, 91, 102, 107–108, 110–111, 115, 117–122, 124, 126, 129, 142, 144, 147–152, 155–159, 168, 171–172, 174–175, 195–198
    viral infectious 72

Arthritis Foundation (AF) 67, 112, 135, 207

arthrocentesis 175

arthrodesis 127–128

arthroscopy 72, 127

Arthrotec 99

arthrotomy 127

artificial tears 69, 91

aspirin 26, 28, 37, 74, 94, 117, 120–121, 150, 152, 162–166, 186

Atabrine 121, 149

auranofin 154

Aurolate 121, 148, 154

autoantibodies xvii, 24, 30, 68, 91, 196

Learn About Your Arthritis!

Learn About Your Arthritis!

T

Learn About Your Arthritis!